Self-Assessment Color Review of

Small Animal Orthopedics

Daniel D. Lewis
DVM, Dipl ACVS
Associate Professor of Small Animal Surgery
University of Florida, Gainesville, Florida, USA

Robert B. Parker
DVM, Dipl ACVS
Chairman and Chief of the Department of Surgery
The Animal Medical Center, New York, New York, USA

Mark S. Bloomberg
DVM, MS, Dipl ACVS
Formerly Collins Professor and Chairman
University of Florida, Gainesville, Florida, USA

Iowa State University Press/Ames

First published in the United States of America in 1998 by
Iowa State University Press, 2121 South State Avenue, Ames, Iowa 50014-8300.
ISBN 0-8138-2947-X
Library of Congress Cataloging-in-Publication Data applied for.

Project management: Paul Bennett
Editor: Peter H. Beynon
Cover design: Patrick Daly
Book design: Dominique Mann
Color reproduction: Reed Digital, Ipswich, UK
Printed by: Grafos SA, Barcelona, Spain

This book is dedicated to

Mark S. Bloomberg
1945–1996

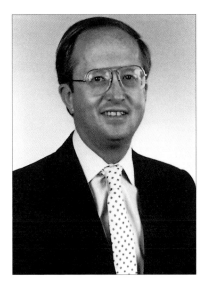

A friend, a colleague, and an inspiration

Acknowledgements

The editors would like to thank Debby A. Sundstrom, Kimberly L. Johnson, Linda S. Lee, and Linda F. Rose for their efforts in preparing the text and illustrations for this book.

The treatment protocol for the radial fracture given in 180, 181 has been used by Dr. Richard Eaton-Wells of Queensland, Australia, on a large number of racing Greyhounds with very good results. The goal is to return these dogs to competitive racing by 16–20 weeks following injury.

Permission was given for the following figures to be reproduced in the book (identified by question numbers):

8b, 159b Previously published in *Compendium of Continuing Education* **17**, 35–49, 1995.

17a–c Previously published in *Journal of the American Animal Hospital Association* **29**(2), 134–40, 1993.

29c Previously published in *Journal of the American Veterinary Medical Association* **208**, 81–4, 1994.

58b, c Previously published in *Small Animal Orthopaedics*, Ed. M.L. Olmstead (1995) Mosby.

67 Previously published in *An Atlas of Veterinary Surgery*, 3rd edn, Eds. Hickman J., Houlton J.E.F. and Edwards B. (1995) Blackwells.

91a–d Previously published in *Journal of the American Animal Hospital Association* **27**(2), 171–8, 1993.

96a, b Previously published in *Journal of the American Veterinary Medical Association* **201**(12), 1897–9, 1992.

116a, b, d Previously published in *Journal of the American Veterinary Medical Association* **194**, 1618–25.

116c Previously published in *Veterinary and Comparative Orthopaedics and Traumatology* **2**, 104–7, 1988.

174a–c Previously published in *Veterinary Surgery* **17**, 128–34, 1988.

Preface

The past decade has seen numerous advancements in the field of small animal ortho-pedics, not only in the basic sciences; the clinical application of imaging modalities, such as computed tomography, magnetic resonance imaging, and scintigraphy; con-tinued experimental and clinical research in biomechanics, cartilage physiology and pathophysiology, bone biology, fracture healing, and musculoskeletal tumor develop-ment and treatment; but also in the technological development of new or improved instrumentation and implant systems, which have greatly enhanced our understanding of orthopedics and the treatment of dogs and cats with orthopedic abnormalities.

This book is not intended to be a comprehensive text reviewing every facet of small animal orthopedics. Rather this book is designed to be an illustrated, self-directed educational tool containing current information which should be of value to veterinary students, interns and residents in training, small animal practitioners with a specific interest in orthopedics, and specialists involved in small animal orthopedics. The broad classification of cases on page 8 allows the reader who is interested in a general aspect of the subject to turn quickly and easily to questions on a related topic, while the index allows the reader to search for a particular subject if desired.

The clinical practice of orthopedics is a combination of science, experience, and judgement. The reader's answers to selected questions may differ from those contained within this book. The contributors have made a thorough effort to make the informa-tion in this book as up to date and accurate as possible, but the reader should be aware that alternative answers to some questions, particularly clinical scenarios, may, and do, exist.

This text is one in a series of self-assessment guides designed to facilitate learning through selected clinical case situations or specific, applied-research materials. An inter-national group of forty-nine orthopedic surgeons, radiologists, pathologists, and anat-omists have contributed to this text. The breadth of their expertise has made the con-tent of this text diverse, in-depth, and on the cutting edge of small animal orthopedics.

This book was inspired by the late Mark S. Bloomberg. The contributors enthusiasti-cally gave their time in their desire to pay respect to a man who influenced us all as veterinarians, surgeons, and individuals. We hope this book will serve its readers as a valuable learning tool.

Daniel D. Lewis
Robert B. Parker
April 1998

Contributors

A. Rick Alleman, DVM, PhD,
Dipl ABVP and ACVP
University of Florida, Gainesville,
Florida, USA

Mark A. Anderson, DVM, MS,
Dipl ACVS
University of Pennsylvania, Philadelphia,
Pennsylvania, USA

Dennis N. Aron, DVM, Dipl ACVS
University of Georgia, Athens, Georgia,
USA

Jamie R. Bellah, DVM, Dipl ACVS
University of Florida, Gainesville,
Florida, USA

Christopher R. Bellenger, BVSc, MVB,
PhD, FACVSc, MRCVS, Dipl ECVS
University College Dublin, Ballsbridge,
Dublin, Ireland

Scott G. Bertrand, DVM, Dipl ACVS
Dallas Veterinary Surgical Center,
Dallas, Texas, USA

Jean-Pierre Cabassu, DV, Dipl ECVS
Clinique Veterinaire, Marseille, France

Alan R. Cross, DVM, Dipl ACVS
University of Florida, Gainsville,
Florida, USA

Jacek J. deHaan, DVM, Dipl ACVS and
ECVS
Affiliated Veterinary Specialists,
Winter Park, Florida, USA

Gary W. Ellison, DVM, MS, Dipl ACVS
University of Florida, Gainesville,
Florida, USA

Randall B. Fitch, DVM, MS, Dipl ACVS
Louisiana State University, Baton Rouge,
Louisiana, USA

John P. Graham, MVB, MSc, DVR,
MRCVS, Dipl ACVR and ECVDI
University of Florida, Gainsville,
Florida, USA

Robin H. Holtsinger, DVM, Dipl ACVS
Fort Lauderdale, Florida, USA

John E.F. Houlton, MA, VetMB, DVR,
DSAO, MRCVS, Dipl ECVS
University of Cambridge, Cambridge, UK

Donald A. Hulse, DVM, Dipl ACVS
Texas A & M University, College
Station, Texas, USA

Ann L. Johnson, DVM, MS, Dipl ACVS
University of Illinois, Urbana, Illinois,
USA

Kenneth A. Johnson, MVSc, PhD,
MRCVS, FACVSc, Dipl ACVS and
ECVS
University of Bristol, Bristol, Avon, UK

Sharon C. Kerwin, DVM, MS, Dipl ACVS
Louisiana State University, Baton Rouge,
Louisiana, USA

Otto I. Lanz, DVM
University of Florida, Gainesville,
Florida, USA

Daniel D. Lewis, DVM, Dipl ACVS
University of Florida, Gainesville,
Florida, USA

Diane T. Lewis, DVM, Dipl ACVD
University of Florida, Gainesville,
Florida, USA

Darryl E. McDonald, DVM, MS,
Dipl ACVS
Dallas Veterinary Surgical Center,
Dallas, Texas, USA

Ronald M. McLaughlin, Jr., DVM,
DVSc, Dipl ACVS
Kansas State University, Manhattan,
Kansas, USA

G. Craig MacPherson, BVSc, MVSc,
FACVSc
Northern Sydney Small Animal Surgical
Referral Service, Sydney, New South
Wales, Australia

Mark D. Markel, DVM, PhD,
  Dipl ACVS
University of Wisconsin–Madison,
Madison, Wisconsin, USA

Scott T. Murphy, DVM, Dipl ACVS
University of Florida, Gainesville,
Florida, USA

Matt G. Oakes, DVM, Dipl ACVS
Tampa Bay Veterinary Surgery, Largo,
Florida, USA

Maura G. O'Brien, DVM, Dipl ACVS
VCA West Los Angeles Animal Hospital,
Los Angeles, California, USA

Robert B. Parker, DVM, Dipl ACVS
The Animal Medical Center, New York,
New York, USA

Robert D. Pechman, DVM, Dipl ACVR
Louisiana State University, Baton Rouge,
Louisiana, USA

Robert T. Pernell, DVM, MS,
  Dipl ACVS
Costal Carolina Veterinary Surgery,
North Charleston, South Carolina, USA

Steve W. Petersen, DVM, Dipl ACVS
Alameda East Veterinary Hospital,
Denver, Colorado, USA

Alessandro Piras, DVM, DISVS
ARGOS Small Animal Veterinary Clinic,
Collecchio, Parma, Italy

Robert M. Radasch, DVM, MS,
  Dipl ACVS
Dallas Veterinary Surgical Center,
Dallas, Texas, USA

Richard A. Read, BVSc, PhD, FACVSc
Murdoch University, Murdoch, Western
Australia, Australia

Simon C. Roe, BVSc, MS, PhD,
  Dipl ACVS
North Carolina State University,
Raleigh, North Carolina, USA

G. Diane Shelton, DVM, PhD,
  Dipl ACVIM
University of California, San Diego,
California, USA

Peter K. Shires, BVSc, MS, Dipl ACVS
Virginia Tech, Blacksburg, Virginia, USA

Jonathan T. Shiroma, DVM, MS,
  Dipl ACVR
MedVet, Columbus, Ohio, USA

Gail K. Smith, VMD, PhD
University of Pennsylvania, Philadelphia,
Pennsylvania, USA

Mark M. Smith, VMD, Dipl ACVS
Virginia Tech, Blacksburg, Virginia, USA

Jeffrey T. Stallings, DVM, Dipl ACVS
Chesapeake Veterinary Referral Center,
Annapolis, Maryland, USA

W. Preston Stubbs, DVM, Dipl ACVS
Massey University, Palmerston North,
New Zealand

Geoff. Sumner-Smith, BVSc, MS,
  DVSc (Liv), FRCVS
University of Guelph, Guelph, Ontario,
Canada

Henri J.J. van Bree, DVM, PhD,
  Dipl ECVS, Dipl ECVDI
University of Ghent, Merelbeke, Belgium

Rene T. Van Ee, DVM, Dipl ACVS
Sheridan Animal Hospital, Buffalo, New
York, USA

Kirk L. Wendleberg, DVM, Dipl ACVS
Animal Specialty Group, Los Angeles,
California, USA

J. Carroll Woodard, DVM, PhD,
  Dipl ACVP
University of Florida, Gainesville,
Florida, USA

Thomas J. Wronski, PhD
University of Florida, Gainesville,
Florida, USA

Broad classification of cases

Abbreviations

ATP Adenosine triphosphate
bid *Bis in die* (twice a day)
CCL Cranial cruciate ligament
DCP Dynamic compression plate
EMG Electromyography
GC Glucocorticoid
H & E Hematoxylin and eosine (stain)
HO Hypertrophic osteopathy
HOD Hypertrophic osteodystrophy

NSAIDs Non-steroidal anti-inflammatory drugs
OCD Osteochondritis dissecans
OFA Orthopedic Foundation for Animals
PMMA Polymethylmethacrylate
po *Per os* (by mouth)
PSGAGs Polysulfated glycosaminoglycans
RCC Retained cartilage core

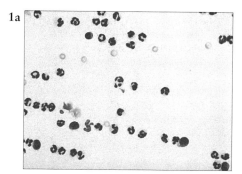
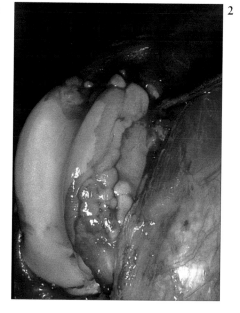

1a   1b

1 A four-year-old, intact male Doberman Pinscher was presented with bilateral carpal joint effusion. Radiographs revealed soft tissue swelling, but no degenerative or erosive changes. Synovial fluid obtained from each carpal joint had a similar cytologic appearance (1a, b). The nucleated cell count was $32 \times 10^9/l$ and the viscosity was decreased.
i. What are the landmarks for arthrocentesis of the carpus?
ii. Give a cytologic description and interpretation of the abnormalities.
iii. Discuss possible etiologies.

2 An intraoperative photograph of the trochlear ridges of the femoral condyle which have been exposed by a medial arthrotomy and lateral dislocation of the patella (2).
i. What are the pathologic structures present on the trochlear ridges?
ii. Describe, on a microstructural level, how these structures develop.

2

9

1 i. Arthrocentesis of the carpus is best approached on the cranial aspect of the limb. The most accessible site is the radiocarpal joint space. With the carpus slightly flexed, a depression can be felt on the craniomedial aspect of the articulation between the distal radius and the proximal radiocarpal bone. The needle should be inserted perpendicular at this point of entry.

ii. The background is lightly granular and eosinophilic indicating decreased mucin content of the synovial fluid. The nucleated cell population consists of predominantly non-degenerate neutrophils containing nuclei with dark chromatin and clear cytoplasm. A single lymphocyte is also present (**1b**). Infectious agents are not visualized.

The interpretation would be non-septic, inflammatory joint disease. Normal synovial fluid in dogs should contain less than 3×10^9 nucleated cells/l, the vast majority of which should be mononuclear cells (lymphocytes, monocytes, macrophages and an occasional synovial lining cell). Normal joint fluid contains few (<10%) neutrophils. A predominant population of neutrophils (50%) indicates inflammatory joint disease. Radiographic analysis is required to distinguish between erosive and non-erosive inflammatory joint disease.

iii. The absence of erosive changes on radiographs, along with the cytologic appearance of non-septic, inflammatory joint fluid is typical of immune-mediated joint disease. Immune-mediated joint disease can be due to antibodies directed against tissues of the joint, or deposition of circulating immune complexes in synovial membranes. Conditions such as idiopathic polyarthritis, systemic lupus erythematosus and drug induced polyarthritis (e.g. sulfamethoxazole–trimethoprim compounds) should be considered as possible etiologies. Immune complex deposition may also be secondary to chronic infections such as septicemia, pyometra, pyorrhea or heartworm disease. Infectious agents such as *Ehrlichia* spp. and *Borrelia* spp. may also infect joints directly but may not cause the erosive joint disease typically seen with septic arthritis. Organisms may or may not be identified cytologically in the synovial fluid. This dog was being treated for a bacterial pyoderma with a sulfamethoxazole–trimethoprim compound. The dog's clinical signs subsided once the drug was discontinued.

2 i. There is extensive osteophyte development along the abaxial surfaces of the trochlear ridges.

ii. Osteophytes develop in response to inflammation of the synovial tissues. Osteophytes develop primarily at the junction of the synovium and bone. When the synovium becomes inflamed, non-specific mutogenic factors are present within the fluid and the capsular tissues. Vascularity increases to the joint as a whole. Cells adjacent to bone proliferate and appear to be directed along the chondrogenic/osteogenic pathway of differentiation rather than the fibrogenic path, as occurs in the rest of the capsule. The fact that osteophytes are derived from tissue adjacent to bone or the proximity of bone matrix itself may be influencing factors. Continued presence of stimulatory factors leads to matrix deposition, mineralization and growth of osteophytes. Once established, osteophyte expansion may also proceed by surface growth. The mineralized areas develop a trabecular architecture and often retain a cartilage surface. Mature osteophytes may become incorporated into the metaphyseal trabecular structure during remodeling.

3 Identify the regions or points labeled a–d in the load/deformation curve shown (3).

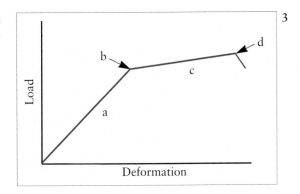

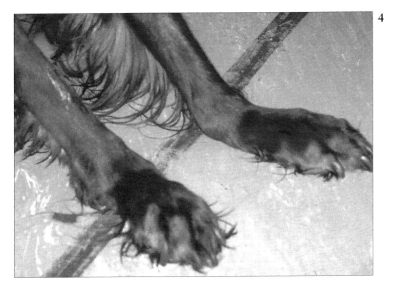

4 A photograph of the distal forelimb of a dog that jumped from a 6 m height and acutely developed this deformity (4).
i. What is the most likely diagnosis?
ii. What pathology is typically associated with this condition?
iii. What radiographic view should be obtained prior to surgical treatment of this conditon?

3, 4: Answers

3 The most important mechanical qualities of a structure are its stiffness and strength. Under the influence of externally applied forces, or loads, a structure deforms or changes in dimensions. When a load in a known direction is imposed on a structure, the deformation of the structure can be measured and recorded on a load/deformation curve. The load/deformation curve is useful for determining the mechanical properties of whole structures such as whole bone or bone implant composites. The initial straight portion of the curve (a) is the *elastic region*. This portion of the curve defines the elasticity of a structure. As load is applied in the elastic region, deformation occurs but is not permanent; the structure returns to its original shape after the load is removed. If, however, loading continues, the outermost fibers of the structure begin to yield, defining the *yield point* (b) beyond which the structure will not return to its original shape after the load is removed, i.e. the structure will have some residual deformation. This region of the curve beyond the yield point (c) is known as the *plastic region*. If loading is increased, the structure will eventually fail, defining the *ultimate failure point* (d). The stiffness of the structure can be determined from the slope of the load/deformation curve in the elastic region. The steeper the slope, the stiffer the structure. Three parameters for determining the strength of a structure can be determined from the load/deformation curve. These include the load the structure can withstand before failing, the deformation the structure can withstand before failing, and the energy the structure can absorb before failing. The strength, either in load or deformation, known as the ultimate strength, can be determined from the curve by the ultimate failure point. The strength in terms of energy storage is determined by the magnitude of the area under the entire curve. The larger the area, the higher the energy storage before failure.

4 i. Bilateral carpal hyperextension injuries.
ii. The palmar support for the carpus is derived from a myriad of small ligaments that support the surrounding bones and fibrocartilage. A major misconception is that carpal hyperextension injuries are caused by flexor tendon disruption. The tendon of insertion of the flexor carpi radialis muscle contributes minimally to the stability of the carpus. The main structure supporting the palmar aspect of the antebrachiocarpal joint is a complex of ligaments which connect the distal radius, the distal ulna and the accessory carpal bone to the palmar aspect of the radial carpal bone. The intercarpal joint is also supported by an array of small, unnamed ligaments. The carpometacarpal joint is supported by the strong palmar carpal fibrocartilage, many small ligaments and two strong accessory carpal-metacarpal ligaments. Hyperextension injuries result from disruption of some or all of these anatomic structures.
iii. In addition to dorsopalmar and lateral view radiographs, stress radiographs should be obtained to establish the level(s) of the instability. Stress radiographs are necessary to identify the location of the instability. Standing, cross-table radiographs are obtained with the dog weight-bearing (lifting the ipsilateral limb will increase weight-bearing) using a horizontal beam. If instability is confined to the intracarpal and carpometacarpal joint, a partial carpal arthrodesis may be indicated; however, if there is instability of the antebrachiocarpal joint, a pancarpal arthrodesis should be considered.

5 A 12-month-old, intact female German Shepherd Dog is being screened for hip dysplasia using the standard ventrodorsal hip extended radiographic view.
i. Describe the Orthopedic Foundation for Animals (OFA) criteria, calculation of the Norberg angle and the distraction–stress method (PennHIP) for evaluating and diagnosing canine hip dysplasia.
ii. What coxofemoral joint structure has been shown to mask joint laxity when a dog's coxofemoral joints are positioned for standard ventrodorsal hip extended view radiographs?

6a
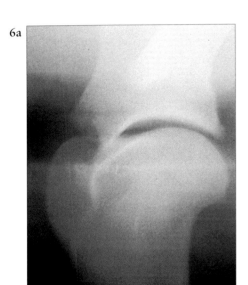

6b
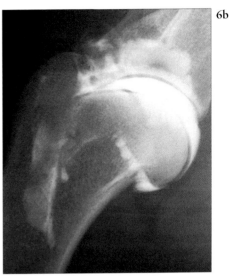

6 Plain mediolateral view radiograph (6a), positive-contrast arthrogram (6b) and arthroscopic view (6c) of the scapulohumeral joint of a two-year-old Bernese Mountain Dog with a right forelimb lameness of one year's duration. Describe the radiographic, arthrographic and arthroscopic abnormalities, and define the final diagnosis.

6c
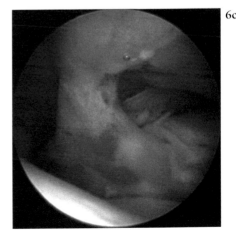

5a

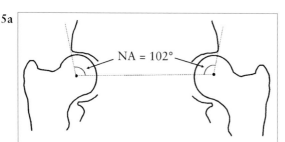

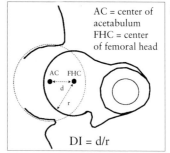

5b

AC = center of acetabulum
FHC = center of femoral head

DI = d/r

5 i. Using the OFA seven point scoring system (excellent, good, fair, borderline, mild hip dysplasia, moderate hip dysplasia and severe hip dysplasia), a subjective score is used to evaluate hip laxity and degenerative joint diseases. In contrast, two quantitative methods have been developed to determine passive hip laxity. The Norberg angle (NA) method quantitates hip laxity from a standard hip extended radiographic projection. The Norberg angle is calculated as the angle defined by or formed by lines that intersect at the center of the femoral head. The first line is one connecting the center of each femoral head and the other line is drawn from the center of the femoral head to the craniodorsal acetabular rim (5a). Norberg angles less than 105° are considered abnormal and indicative of dysplasia. The distraction–stress method is based on the relative degree of femoral head displacement from the acetabulum (DI = d/r where d is equal to the distance from the center of the acetabulum to the center of the femoral head and r is the radius of the femoral head) which is measured on the distraction view (5b). Measured values are used to formulate a distraction index (DI). A fully congruent hip would have an index of 0 and a fully luxated hip would have an index of 1 or greater.

ii. As the coxofemoral joint is placed in extreme extension, the joint capsule tightens due to tensioning of the spiral fibrous elements of the capsule. Joint capsule tightening not only limits further extension, but may act to seat the femoral head into the acetabulum, masking joint laxity. This may explain the poor sensitivity of the standard ventrodorsal radiography to define inherent joint laxity. The neutral distraction position of the coxofemoral joint has been shown to assess passive hip laxity and be four times more sensitive in detecting passive hip laxity when compared with the standard ventrodorsal hip extended position.

6 There is an irregularity of the supraglenoid tubercle and calcification in the origin of the biceps brachii tendon on the plain radiographs. The positive-contrast arthrogram fails to demonstrate the attachment of the biceps brachii tendon, which is normally visible as a band-like filling defect within the bicipital tendon sheath. Leakage of contrast medium is also visible in this same area. Distension of the scapulohumeral joint due to inflammatory changes is also visible. No radiographic abnormalities suggestive of osteochondrosis are present. The arthroscopic view shows that the attachment of the bicipital tendon sheath on the supraglenoid tubercle is nearly completely disrupted. This dog has a partial rupture of the tendon of origin of the biceps brachii muscle and severe synovitis.

7 With regard to the two-year-old Bernese Mountain Dog in 6:
i. What is the etiopathogenesis of the condition?
ii. What is the proposed treatment?

8 A drawing of an external skeletal fixator used to stabilize a comminuted tibial fracture with a concurrent segmental fracture of the ipsilateral fibula (8a).
i. Give a technical description of this external skeletal fixator configuration.
ii. Under what circumstances is this configuration typically used in dogs?

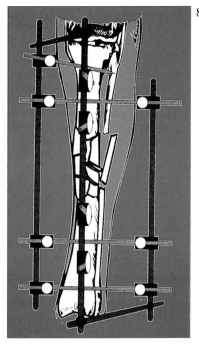

8a

9 A photograph of the mouth of a cat which has undergone a stabilization procedure for a comminuted fracture of the angle of the left mandible (9).
i. What form of stabilization has been utilized?
ii. How should the canine teeth be prepared for this procedure?

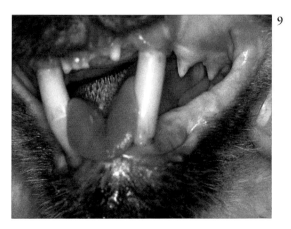

9

15

7 i. Although a traumatic origin should be considered, this partial rupture is probably a sequela to bicipital tenosynovitis. In this particular dog these findings were bilateral, which supports this theory. Bicipital tenosynovitis is often associated with OCD of the humeral head but in this dog there are no radiographic abnormalities suggestive of osteochondrosis.

ii. This lesion should be treated by transection of the bicipital tendon at its origin and reattachment of the tendon to the greater tubercle of the humerus by use of a screw and spiked washer. In this dog, severance of the tendon was done arthroscopically, which caused minimal soft tissue trauma.

8 i. A bilateral–biplanar (type III) fixator configuration (or montage) constructed by articulating a unilateral–uniplanar (type I) frame with a bilateral–uniplanar (type II) frame. Two articulations are used in this montage, one from the proximocranial connector to the proximomedial connector and the other from the distocranial connector to the distolateral connector

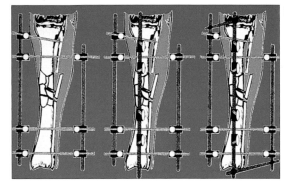

8b

(8b). The articulations 'tie-in' the two separate frames together so that the montage performs as an unit.

ii. Type III configurations are used principally to stabilize mechanically and biologically complex fractures of the radius and ulna or the tibia and fibula. Mechanically, this fracture reconstruction does not result in load sharing through the bone column. Biologically, slow healing is expected because there is typically substantial soft tissue damage associated with highly comminuted fractures. In fracture reconstructions with poor load sharing and substantial soft tissue damage, this highly stable configuration is necessary to maintain stability of the fracture and a firm fixation pin–bone interface resulting in low patient morbidity. Close proximity of the humerus to the thorax and the femur to the trunk precludes application of bilateral frames for humeral or femoral fractures in dogs and cats.

9 i. Columns of dental composite have been used to bond the ipsilateral mandibular and maxillary canine teeth. Bonding of the canine teeth is a non-invasive means of stabilizing mandibular fractures.

ii. The teeth should be cleaned with an ultrasonic scaler and pumiced. The canine teeth are then acid etched, rinsed and dried with a blow dryer. A thin layer of dental adhesive is then applied to the canine teeth. The fracture is held in reduction and the composite is applied. In this cat, plastic drinking straws were filled with composite material to form the columns. The fracture must be held in reduction until the composite has cured. A primary concern is that the repair will eventually lead to proper occlusion.

10   With regard to the cat in **9**, what advantages are associated with the use of this technique?

11   A six-year-old Rottweiler presents with a three-week history of non-weight-bearing left hindlimb lameness. There is pain on palpation of the stifle region and slight soft tissue swelling in the area of the proximal tibia. A lateral view radiograph of the affected tibia is shown (**11a**).
i. Describe the radiographic abnormalities.
ii. Give a differential diagnosis.
iii. What other diagnostic test should be carried to establish a definitive diagnosis for this dog?

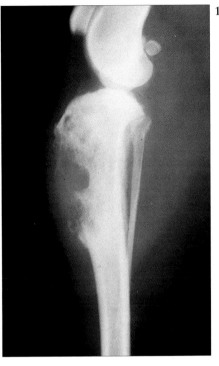
11a

10 The procedure is not invasive and can be performed in a relative short period of time. There is no risk of damaging tooth roots, which can be a complication with many forms of internal and external fixation of mandibular fractures. The animal can eat and drink by itself as the canine teeth are bonded with the mouth partially open. This circumvents the need for pharyngostomy or gastrostomy tube placement. Also, because the canine teeth are bonded with the mouth partially open, the risk of hyperthermia and aspiration is decreased. This technique is particularly useful in cats, brachycephalic breeds of dogs, and animals with poor mandibular bone quality. It does require four salvageable canine teeth.

11 i. A moderately aggressive, predominantly osteolytic, multi-centric lesion involving the proximal tibia. Mild soft tissue swelling is associated with this lesion. The adjacent bones and the stifle joint are radiographically normal.
ii. Must include primary or secondary bone neoplasia, and bacterial or fungal osteomyelitis.
iii. Thoracic radiographs should

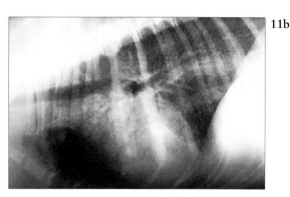
11b

be obtained to search for evidence of metastatic neoplasia or fungal pneumonia. Thoracic radiographs in this dog revealed a diffuse nodular interstitial pattern typically associated with blastomycosis pneumonia (**11b**). Blood should be drawn and submitted for fungal titers. Most importantly, biopsies of the lesion should be obtained for microbiologic culture and histopathologic examination. This dog was found to have fungal osteomyelitis caused by *Blastomyces dermatiditis*. Fungal osteomyelitis may radiographically mimic bone neoplasia. Lesions are most often proliferative in nature, but may occasionally be predominantly osteolytic as in this dog. Coccidioidomycosis, seen in south-western United States, may involve bone in about half of the cases. Other systemic fungi affect bone less commonly. Dogs with fungal osteomyelitis often respond to appropriate medical treatment. A lateral view radiograph of this dog's tibia obtained seven months after appropriate anti-fungal therapy is shown (**11c**).

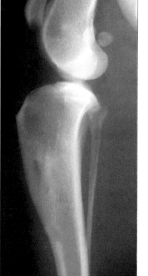
11c

12a 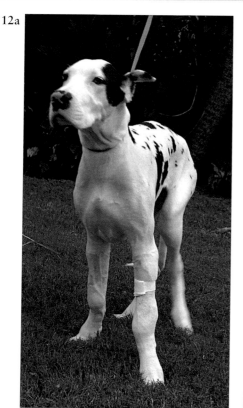 12b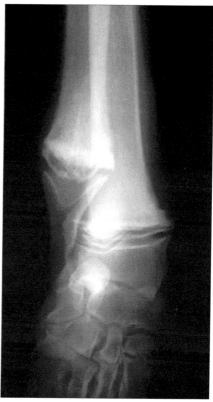

12 A photograph (**12a**) and craniocaudal view radiograph (**12b**) of the right distal antebrachium and carpus of a five-month-old, male Great Dane that is depressed, anorexic, febrile and reluctant to walk.
i. Describe the radiographic abnormalities and state a diagnosis.
ii. What is the etiology of this disease?
iii. What treatment is appropriate for this dog?

13 Discuss the advantages of tracheostomy tube placement in dogs or cats with complex maxillary or mandibular fractures.

12 i. The radiograph reveals an irregular radiolucent zone involving the metaphysis subjacent and parallel to the distal radial and ulnar physes. These radiographic abnormalities are characteristic of early HOD. There is also a small RCC affecting the distal ulna. HOD is an acute suppurative inflammatory disease affecting long bones of rapidly growing, juvenile, large-breed dogs. The radiolucent areas seen radiographically correspond to regions of non-septic suppurative (predominantly non-degenerate neutrophils) inflammation. Metaphyseal trabecular infarction is seen and perimetaphyseal periosteal new bone is evident. The bone scan of the forelimbs in this dog (12c) reveals increased uptake in the regions where non-septic suppurative inflammation and trabecular infarction in the metaphyseal regions is present.

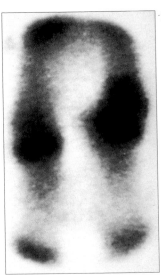

12c

ii. The cause of HOD is unknown. The disease is not heritable. Hypovitaminosis C has been purported as a cause of HOD; however, dogs produce ascorbic acid endogenously and dogs with HOD have normal ascorbic acid levels. Supplementation of ascorbic acid neither resolves nor prevents recurrence of clinical abnormalities. Overnutrition with protein, vitamins such as vitamin D, minerals and energy have all been anecdotally associated with HOD, but experimental oversupplementation of these nutrients has not produced HOD. Correction of potential dietary influences does not alter the course of HOD. Although infectious agents have not been identified histologically or cultured from dogs with HOD, canine distemper virus has been detected in bone cells of dogs with HOD using *in situ* hybridization techniques. The association between HOD and canine distemper virus infection, however, remains speculative.
iii. Treatment of HOD is supportive and directed at maintenance of hydration, nutritional support and prevention of pressure sores. Exercise restriction is recommended to reduce the potential for additional bone infarction. Anti-inflammatory drugs can be prescribed to mitigate pain and pyrexia. Occasionally, a debilitated puppy will not respond and will die or be euthanized. Dogs that recover from HOD may have varying degrees of bone deformity depending on the severity of the disease. Permanent antebrachial bowing deformities associated with attenuated or arrested physeal growth can occur.

13 Placement of a temporary tracheostomy tube pre-operatively provides an unobstructed airway when there is peri-pharyngeal edema and trauma. Patients with respiratory distress breathe more comfortably after this procedure. Tracheostomy intubation allows an unimpeded surgical field during surgical stabilization of maxillary and mandibular fractures as well as accurate assessment of occlusion during fracture reduction and stabilization.

14 A photograph of a dog's stifle joint with advanced degenerative joint disease (14).
i. Why is the administration of PSGAGs considered to be beneficial in the treatment of degenerative joint disease?
ii. How should PSGAGs be administered?

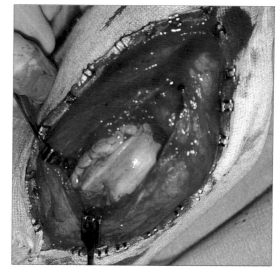

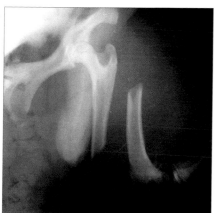

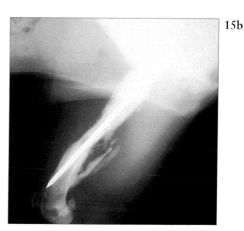

15 A five-year-old Golden Retriever became non-weight-bearing and developed a serosanguinous discharge from a fistulous tract which opened dorsal to the greater trochanter of the femur six weeks following surgical repair of a femoral fracture. Pre-operative (15a) and six weeks post-operative (15b) radiographs are shown.
i. What is the tentative diagnosis?
ii. What diagnostic test(s) could be used to help support or refute the tentative diagnosis?
iii. What could have been done to prevent this complication?

14 i. PSGAGs are classified as disease-modifying anti-osteoarthritis drugs and are often referred to as chondroprotective agents. While evidence for active production of cartilage matrix is less certain, PSGAGs do inhibit proteinases which would otherwise accelerate matrix destruction. Cartilage destruction associated with degenerative joint disease can result from the direct action of serine proteinases such as elastase and cathepsin G, extracellular metalloproteinases such as stromelysin and collagenase, or lysozomal enzymes including hyaluronidase on proteoglycan and collagen. PSGAGs have been shown to ameliorate the degradative effects of such enzymes on articular cartilage *in vitro*. The negatively charged sulfate groups on PSGAGs are thought to interact with the positively charged amino acid residues on proteins, including the neutral metalloproteinases. PSGAGs stimulate production of hyaluronic acid by synoviocytes and also have a fibrinolytic effect which is thought to improve synovial and subchondral bone circulation. Some PSGAGs also induce superoxide dismutase production which may scavenge superoxide radicals.

In dogs in which the CCL was transected, concentrations of collagenase in the cartilage of PSGAG-treated dogs were less than in untreated dogs. Administration of PSGAGs has also been shown to decrease active neutral metalloproteinase concentrations in cartilage following partial medial meniscectomy. In a double-blind clinical trial including 40 dogs with osteoarthritis, weekly subcutaneous administration of PSGAGs (3 mg/kg) for four weeks resulted in a favorable response over placebo treatment in regard to lameness, body condition, pain on joint manipulation and willingness to exercise.

ii. PSGAGs cross the synovial membrane after subcutaneous and intramuscular injection and accumulate in articular cartilage, menisci and ligaments. The highly negatively charged PSGAGs accumulate preferentially in damaged or inflamed joints. Subcutaneous and intramuscular injection also avoids the risk of hemarthrosis. Intra-articular injection of PSGAGs lowers the minimum number of bacterial organisms needed to establish infection in a joint and has been associated with septic arthritis in horses.

15 i. An infected, hypertrophic non-union fracture of the right femur with bone sequestration.

ii. Cytology in addition to aerobic and anaerobic culture and anti-microbial sensitivity from samples obtained from deep aspiration at the fracture site. Samples taken from the fistulous tract often do not accurately reflect the pathogenic organisms present at the fracture site.

iii. Inadequate stability of the fracture in combination with iatrogenic contamination at the time of surgery is the likely cause of this complication. A fracture will heal even if contaminated as long as rigid stability has been provided. Had a more rigid form of stabilization, such as a plate and screws, an intramedullary interlocking nail and screws, or an adjunctive external fixator in conjunction with the intramedullary pin, been used initially, the non-union and possibly the osteomyelitis would not have occurred. The configuration of this fracture was not amenable to repair with an intramedullary pin and cerclage wire alone.

16 With regard to the Golden Retriever with the infected non-union fracture in **15**, describe how this case should be managed.

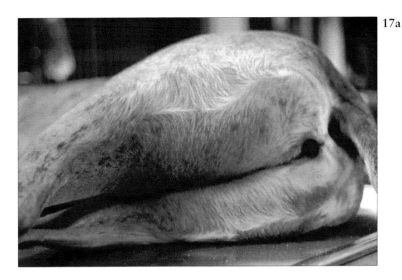

17a

17 Compartment syndrome is most commonly associated with trauma, vascular injury or post-operative complications. A photograph of a three-year-old, female Greyhound that sustained a left femur fracture and has compartment syndrome is shown (**17a**).
i. Briefly define the pathophysiologic and anatomic basis of compartment syndrome.
ii. Name the four anatomic locations in which compartment syndrome has been experimentally produced in dogs.
iii. What is the objective diagnostic procedure used to identify this condition?
iv. What is the treatment for this condition?

16 Infected non-union fractures require surgical intervention. Antibiotics alone will not resolve the infection. The sequestra should be surgically removed and the involucrum debrided until well-vascularized tissue is exposed. Appropriate culture specimens should be obtained at surgery. All implants should be removed and a more rigid form of fixation, such as a bone plate, an interlocking intramedullary nail or an external fixator, used. Fresh autogenous cancellous bone graft should be placed at the fracture site to stimulate bone production, decrease dead space and enhance vascularity. Delayed cancellous grafting may be considered. The surgical wound can either be closed primarily and a low-vacuum closed suction system implanted, or delayed closure can be performed when healthy granulation tissue is present. The dog should be placed on prolonged antimicrobial therapy based on the results of the culture and sensitivity. Once the fracture has healed, all metallic implants should be removed to eradicate the infection.

17 i. Regional neuromuscular ischemia due to elevated pressure within a defined anatomic space. The elevated pressure is usually due to hemorrhage or increased blood flow into the space. When barriers to swelling are bone and fascia, the condition is termed osteofascial compartment syndrome.

ii. Craniolateral compartment of the crus; caudal compartment of the crus; caudal compartment of the antebrachium; femoral compartment (this is a multifascial compartment with three distinct fascial envelopes: the quadriceps mechanism; the hamstring group; and the adductor muscle).

iii. Compartmental pressures can be objectively measured using a wick catheter, a slit catheter or an 18 gauge hollow-bore needle and a saline-filled central venous pressure manometer (**17b**). This dog's femoral compartment pressure exceeded 25 mmHg. Compartment pressures in normal dogs range from -2.0–8.0 mmHg. In most cases, tissue pressure within the affected compartment remains below diastolic blood pressure; therefore, the presence of palpable peripheral pulses, normal capillary refill time and pink color of the distal extremity cannot be used to exclude the existence of a compartment syndrome.

iv. Surgical decompression of the involved compartments with fasciotomy if compartment pressures exceed 30 mmHg. A fasciotomy was performed in this dog (**17c**) and the left hindlimb was packed with ice following surgery. The femoral fracture was repaired five days later when the femoral compartment pressure had returned to normal.

18 A photograph of a two-year-old, male Siamese cat that has a weight-bearing lameness of the right forelimb of three months' duration (18a). The right scapula can be seen to displace dorsally when weight is placed on the right forelimb.
i. What is the diagnosis?
ii. How should this cat be treated?

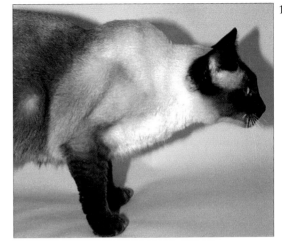

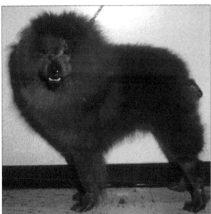

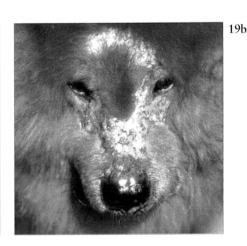

19 Photographs of a one-year-old, male Chow Chow with multifocal scarring alopecia; hyperpigmentation and ulceration of the face, tail tip and distal extremities; and a stiff gait in all four limbs (19a, b). There is muscle atrophy of the temporal and triceps muscles. The dog's skin lesions have been present since six months of age.
i. What is the most likely diagnosis?
ii. What diagnostic tests should be considered to confirm the diagnosis?
iii. Assuming the diagnosis is correct, what is the prognosis?

18 i. Dorsal luxation of the scapula. Dorsal luxation of the scapula is associated with avulsion or tearing of the serratus ventralis, rhomboideus and trapezius muscles. The muscles are usually torn at or near their insertions on the cranial angle and caudal border of the scapula allowing the scapula to displace dorsally during weight-bearing.

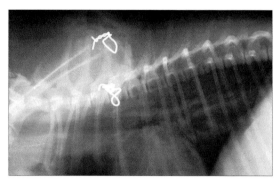

18b

ii. Dorsal luxation of the scapula is a traumatic injury usually associated with jumping or falling from a height. Although the resultant gait abnormality is generally well-tolerated by dogs and cats, surgical intervention is necessary to resolve the lameness. A caudodorsal approach to the scapula exposes the serratus ventralis, rhomboideus and trapezius muscles, and an attempt should be made to suture these muscles primarily. This repair is generally weak and tenuous, and therefore all muscular repairs are supported with orthopedic wires passed through two holes drilled in the caudal portion of the body of the scapula and around an adjacent rib (**18b**). The limb should be placed in a Velpeau sling or spica splint for two to three weeks following surgery.

19 i. Dermatomyositis, which has been observed in Collies, Shetland Sheepdogs, Chow Chows, a Pembroke Welsh Corgi and an Australian cattle dog. This disease has an autosomal dominant mode of inheritance in Collies, but the pattern of inheritance has not yet been established in other breeds.
ii. The diagnosis is made based on clinical signs, histologic evaluation of affected muscles and skin, and EMG. Skin lesions usually occur in young dogs; however, skin lesions may be so mild that they are missed at an early age. A skin biopsy of an alopecic, scarred lesion is preferred. Evidence of myositis is present on histologic evaluation of muscle. Fibrillation potentials, positive sharp waves, and bizarre high frequency discharges should be present on EMG of muscles of the head, trunk and extremities of affected dogs.
iii. Disease severity varies widely in dogs with dermatomyositis, making prognosis difficult to predict and therapeutic trials difficult to evaluate. The disease often waxes and wanes of its own accord. Skin lesions of mildly affected dogs may heal without scarring and the dogs may live normal lives. Moderately affected dogs may have cutaneous scarring and some muscle atrophy. More severely affected dogs have persistent skin and muscle disease with stunted growth. Secondary pyoderma, demodicosis and aspiration pneumonia from involvement of esophageal muscles are potential problems in severely affected dogs. Therapy with vitamin E, corticosteroids and pentoxifylline has provided variable results.

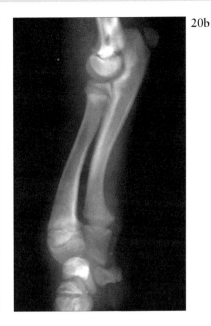

20 Craniocaudal (20a) and lateral (20b) view radiographs of the left antebrachium of a ten-week-old, male Cocker Spaniel with a weight-bearing lameness of the left forelimb.
i. Describe the radiographic abnormalities present.
ii. What will be the likely result if this dog is not treated?
iii. What would be the appropriate treatment for this dog?

21 A photograph of an 11-month-old Weimaraner that had a distal left femoral fracture stabilized with a single intramedullary pin when it was six months of age (21). The dog was placed in a full limb cast four weeks following surgery. The left stifle is now fixed in hyperextension. What syndrome is affecting this dog's stifle?

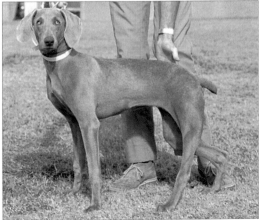

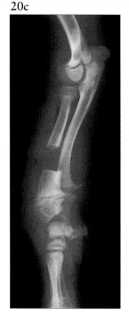

20c

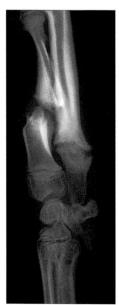

20d

20 i. The distal physis of the left radius is narrow and irregular. There is a dorsal-to-palmar bowing deformity originating at the distal radial physis. The distal radial epiphysis is abnormally shaped and the dorsal cortex is overgrowing the palmar cortex resulting in malalignment of the left radiocarpal joint. The distal radial epiphysis is also displaced medially. The elbow is normal. These radiographic abnormalities are consistent with eccentric, premature closure of the distal physis of the left radius, most likely the result of trauma. The left radius was measured to be approximately 10% shorter than the right radius.

ii. The limb deformity is likely to increase in severity because the dog still has substantial potential for long bone growth. The distal ulnar physis will continue to grow but the radius will restrict normal growth of the antebrachium. The mid-diaphysis of the ulna may bow laterally resulting in a varus carpal deformity. Some internal rotation of the carpus may also develop. In a dog such as this, in which the distal radial physis closes at such a young age, distal subluxation of the radial head often develops. This results in abnormal development of the elbow and degenerative joint disease which can produce substantial lameness.

iii. In a dog of this age, treatment should focus on preventing the deformity from becoming more severe and allowing the ulna to continue to grow without restriction. This can be accomplished by performing a segmental ostectomy of the radius. The periosteum at the ostectomy site must be resected or reflected and sewn over the ends of the bone segments to prevent union of the radius. A free autogenous fat graft can also be placed in the ostectomy site to help prevent union from occurring. In this dog a radial ostectomy, periosteal excision and a free autogenous fat graft were performed (20c). Six weeks after surgery, union of the radius had not occurred, the antebrachium continued to gain length, the articulation of the radiocarpal joint had improved and the dog's lameness had resolved (20d).

21 'Quadriceps tie-down' or 'quadriceps contracture' is a severe form of fracture disease which can develop following fracture of the femur, particularly fractures of the distal femur in young dogs and cats. Placing this dog in a full limb cast following open reduction and internal stabilization of the fracture predisposed the dog to develop severe fracture disease.

22 A photograph of a five-month-old male Alaskan Malamute with a weight-bearing lameness of the right hindlimb of four weeks' duration (22a). The dog walks with the right hindpaw externally rotated and circumducts the limb without flexing the stifle as it brings the limb forward.
i. What is the most likely diagnosis?
ii. What surgical options are available to treat this condition?

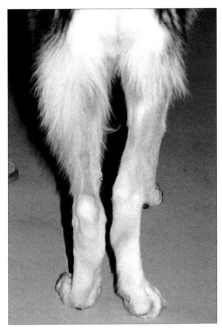

22a

23 Lateral view radiograph of the left distal forelimb of a six-year-old Dober-man Pinscher that had a pancarpal arthrodesis performed previously to treat an open fracture-luxation of the left radius, ulna and carpus (23a). The dog developed lameness and a draining tract over the end of the plate 16 months after the arthrodesis was performed. The plate was removed (23b) and *Staphylococcus intermedius* was cultured from the plate. (The white lines positioned transversely over the limb are radiographic markers in surgical sponges placed over the wound).
What is a cryptic infection?

23a

23b

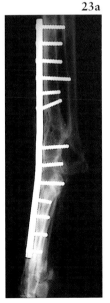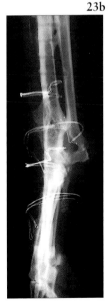

22 i. Lateral patellar luxation is a developmental condition occurring most often in large and giant breed dogs. Dogs with bilateral lateral patellar luxation generally have a crouched hindlimb stance with a knock-kneed (genu valgum) posture. The paws are externally rotated. Coxa valga and an increased angle of anteversion of the coxofemoral joint, an expression of femoral torsion, may be present. These conformational abnormalities result in displacement of the distal femoral shaft towards the midline, away from the normal axis, and increased internal rotation of the distal shaft, thus displacing the femoral trochlea medial to the axis of pull of the quadriceps. Other changes such as a shallow trochlear groove, lateral deviation of the tibial tuberosity and dysplasia of the lateral femoral condyle develop secondary to the altered forces being exerted on the growth plates of the tibia and femur. The medial retinaculum becomes stretched and the lateral retinaculum contracted. The severity of these changes is variable, but in severe cases the skeletal changes can progress rapidly between two and six months of age.

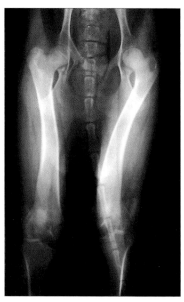

22b

ii. Surgical intervention is recommended. The procedures performed vary with the age of the dog and the severity of the skeletal abnormalities. In very young pups (less than three months) in which the bony abnormalities are minimal, imbrication sutures can be used to support and tighten the medial soft tissues and correct the lateral rotation of the tibia. By placing sutures from the fabella in the medial head of the gastrocnemius muscle to the patella and to the tibial tuberosity, realignment of the quadriceps mechanism can be achieved and the skeletal abnormalities minimized. In this dog, in which skeletal changes are more advanced (**22b**), medial transposition of the tibial tubercle and techniques to deepen the trochlear groove are indicated. Femoral and tibial osteotomies are reserved for severely affected dogs.

23 A latent form of osteomyelitis associated with metallic implants. The causative bacteria are contained in the glycocalyx which is a polysaccharide, mucoid, peribacterial film covering the surface of metallic implants *in vivo*. The glycocalyx prevents antibiotics from reaching the bacteria. The bacteria may stay dormant for years and then unpredictably become active causing signs of localized osteomyelitis. For this reason, removal of all metallic implants used to stabilize infected fractures is advocated once the fracture has healed.

24 A histologic section through a physis stained according to the Von Kossa method with a tetrachrome counterstain (×200) (**24**).
i. Identify the five zones (a–e) of the epiphyseal growth plate.
ii. What are the two most important functions of the growth plate?

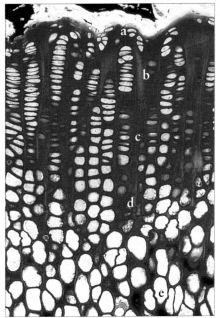

25 A craniocaudal view radiograph of the left elbow of a six-year-old, male Cocker Spaniel that developed an acute non-weight-bearing lameness of the left forelimb while chasing a ball in the owner's yard (**25**).
i. Describe the fracture.
ii. Why are Spaniels predisposed to this particular injury, often as a result of minor trauma?

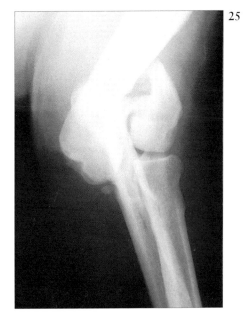

24 i. The growth plate is composed of hyaline cartilage. The different zones of the growth plate are identified based on distinctive, progressive changes in the cartilage cells known as chondrocytes. The thinnest region of the growth plate subjacent to the epiphysis is the zone of resting cells (a). It is composed of relatively few, randomly oriented chondrocytes presumed to function as a cellular reserve. The chondrocytes of the next four zones of the growth plate are arranged in vertical columns parallel to the long axis of the bone. The zone of proliferation (b) is characterized by the presence of many mitotic figures. The chondrocytes here are flattened in appearance and very active in the synthesis and secretion of cartilage matrix. The rapid rate of proliferation of chondrocytes within this zone is primarily responsible for bone elongation. As mitotic activity decreases and the chondrocytes become more ovoid in appearance, the zone of cell maturation (c) is formed. The chondrocytes here are involved mainly in the synthesis and secretion of cartilage matrix. In the zone of cell hypertrophy (d) the chondrocytes become markedly enlarged and vacuolated with swollen, pyknotic nuclei. The cells are located within large lacunar spaces that are separated from adjacent lacunae by thin longitudinal and transverse septae. As the cartilage matrix becomes calcified in the zone of provisional calcification (e), diffusion of nutrients is compromised and the hypertrophic chondrocytes die. Calcified cartilage can be seen as the black-stained areas near the bottom of this figure. Interestingly, the longitudinal septae between the columnar lacunae become well calcified whereas the transverse septae calcify poorly. Consequently, these latter septae are preferentially resorbed by chondroclasts at the junction of the growth plate and metaphysis. The more persistent, calcified longitudinal septae serve as templates for the formation of bone spicules (primary trabeculae) in the primary spongiosa of the metaphysis.
ii. To generate bone elongation and to provide a framework for the formation of trabecular (cancellous) bone.

25 i. There is an intra-articular fracture of the lateral portion of the left humeral condyle (capitulum) extending through the lateral epicondylar crest. The capitulum is displaced proximally.
ii. It has long been recognized that fractures of the humeral condyle often occur with minimal trauma and that humeral condylar fractures frequently occur in Spaniels. A developmental defect of the humeral condyle termed 'incomplete ossification' has been described in Spaniels. As the humeral condyle mineralizes in puppies, the two (capitulum and trochlea) ossification centers should unite at 70 ± 14 days after birth. Their bone architecture should become continuous. In Spaniels the connection between the lateral and medial portions of the humeral condyle may be purely fibrous and contain little or no bone. This weak connection predisposes the condyle to fracture with minimal trauma.

26 With regard to the Cocker Spaniel in 25, what is the prognosis for repair and possible complications?

27a   27b   27c   27d

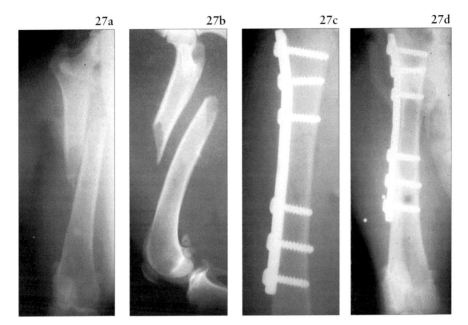

27 Craniocaudal (27a) and lateral (27b) view radiographs of a three-year-old German Shorthaired Pointer that sustained a femoral fracture. The fracture was treated with open reduction and internal fixation with a bone plate (27c). Sixteen-week follow-up craniocaudal (27d) and lateral (27e) view radiographs are shown .

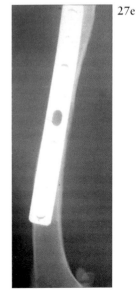

27e

i. What is the predominant type of bone healing occurring in this fracture?
ii. What are the specific requirements for this type of bone healing?

26b

26a
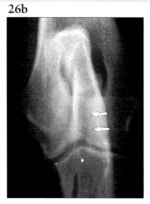

26c
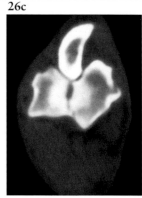

26 The fracture should be anatomically reduced and stabilized with a transcondylar screw placed in lag fashion. In this dog, additional screws were placed in the epicondylar region to provide adjunctive stability (26a). This fracture may not heal because the lateral and medial portions of the condyle were never united. Therefore, the lag screw must provide rigid stabilization for a prolonged period of time. In one case series, 23% of dogs had complications following surgical repair of condylar fractures. The screw may loosen, resulting in pain, or break, resulting in failure of stabilization. When possible, a 4.5 mm cortical bone screw should be selected as this screw has 2.5 times the resistance to bending when compared with a 3.5 mm cortical screw. The contralateral condyle should also be evaluated. If incomplete ossification is present, the potential for fracture of the contralateral condyle exists. A 15° medial oblique craniocaudal view radiograph of the humeral condyle of a two-year-old Brittany is shown (26b). The faint sagittal radiolucent line bisecting the condyle (arrows) is produced by incomplete ossification which was confirmed using computed tomography (26c).

27 i. Primary bone healing in which bone is formed directly between the bone segments without intermediate callus formation. There are two forms of primary bone healing: contact healing and gap healing. Contact healing occurs when fracture surfaces are in direct apposition and is characterized by osteons directly crossing the fracture line. In regions where the fracture segments are not in direct contact but the gap between fracture segments is less than 1 mm, gap healing will occur. In gap healing, lamellar bone is directly formed in the fracture gap without intermediate fibrous or cartilage precursors. The bone is initially deposited perpendicular to the long axis of the bone and is then later remodeled along the lines of functional stress.
ii. There are fundamental biologic, anatomic and biomechanical requirements for primary bone healing to occur. The main biologic requirement is vascularization of the ends of the bone segments. Minimal disruption to adjacent periosteum and soft tissue attachments are also necessary. There must be anatomic reduction resulting in direct apposition of fracture surfaces. Rigid stabilization and interfragmentary compression are the fundamental biomechanical requirements.

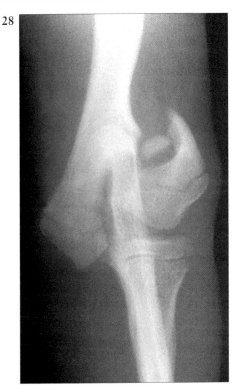

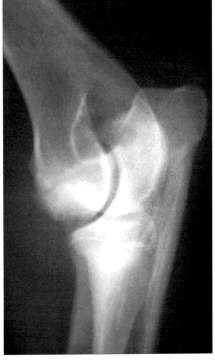

28 A radiograph of the elbow of a five-month-old, male Sharpei that jumped off of the porch and became non-weight-bearing on this limb (28).
i. Describe the Salter–Harris classification scheme for physeal fractures.
ii. What is the Salter–Harris classification of this fracture?

29 An oblique craniocaudal view radio-graph of the right elbow of a ten-month-old, male Labrador Retriever with a right forelimb lameness (29).
i. Describe the radiographic abnormalities.
ii. Describe appropriate surgical treatment of this condition.
iii. List three surgical approaches which would be appropriate for treating this condition and discuss the merits of each approach.

28 The Salter–Harris classification scheme was developed based on the relationship of the fracture line to the growing cells of physis and the radiographic appearance of the fracture. The classification scheme was developed to assist physicians in prognosticating disturbances of continued physeal growth in children. *Type I*: the fracture traverses the physis. *Type II*: the fracture traverses the physis but also involves a portion of the metaphysis. *Type III*: the fracture traverses the physis but also involves a portion of the epiphysis. *Type IV*: the fracture involves a portion of the epiphysis, crosses the physis and also involves a portion of the metaphysis. *Type V*: these are compressive fractures of the physis.

The prognosis for continued growth is favorable with experimentally created type I, II and III fractures. The prognosis for continual growth is less favorable with type IV fractures unless the physis is accurately realigned. Type V injuries are associated with crushing of the cartilagenous growth plate and carry a poor prognosis for continued growth. Unfortunately, the prognostic accuracy of the Salter–Harris classification scheme is not reliable in dogs sustaining traumatically induced physeal fractures. The classification scheme is more useful for describing the radiographic configuration of a particular physeal fracture.

ii. Salter–Harris type IV fracture of the lateral portion of the humeral condyle.

29 i. There are early degenerative changes predominately involving the medial compartment of the elbow joint. There is a subchondral bone defect in the trochlea of the humeral condyle consistent with an osteochondrosis or OCD lesion.

ii. (1) Exploration of the medial compartment of the elbow joint. (2) Excision of the pathologic cartilage. (3) Curettage of the subjacent subchondral bed. (4) The medial coronoid process should also be evaluated as fragmented coronoid process often occurs in association with osteochondrosis/OCD of the humeral condyle.

iii. The medial compartment of the elbow can be approached using either: (1) a proximal ulnar diaphyseal osteotomy. This approach allows visualization of virtually all articular surfaces of the elbow joint but carries substantial post-operative morbidity. The exposure gained with a proximal ulnar diaphyseal osteotomy is rarely warranted and so is not routinely used for dogs with OCD of the humeral condyle or fragmented coronoid process. (2) An osteotomy of the medial epicondyle. This approach allows reflection of the medial collateral ligaments as well as those antebrachial muscles which have their origin on the medial epicondyle. It provides extensive visualization of the medial compartment of the elbow joint, particularly of the trochlea of the humeral condyle, and avoids desmotomy of the medial collateral ligaments; however, complications associated with lag screw stabilization of the osteotomy are frequent. Or (3) a muscle separating approach between the pronator teres and flexor carpi radialis muscles. This approach between the pronator teres and flexor carpi radialis muscles generally affords sufficient exposure for the surgeon to evaluate and treat osteochondritis lesions of the humeral condyle and fragmented coronoid process. Often this approach can be performed without incising the medial collateral ligaments; however, should a desmotomy be required, the clinical morbidity associated with performing a desmotomy is negligible. Arthroscopic treatment has also been described.

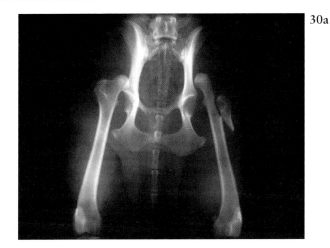

30a

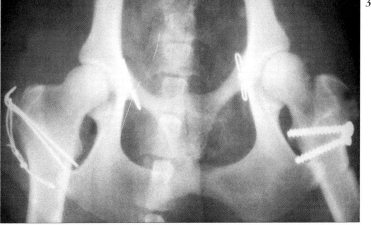

30b

30 Pre-operative (30a) and post-operative (30b) ventrodorsal view radiographs of the pelvis of a six-year-old, 40-kg Labrador Retriever that was hit by a truck.
i. Describe the injuries present.
ii. Describe the surgical procedures used to treat this dog.

31 What centers of ossification are involved in the formation of the acetabulum?

30 i. There is a fracture of the greater trochanter of the left femur and bilateral coxofemoral luxations.
ii. The fracture of the greater trochanter was stabilized with two screws placed in lag fashion. A toggle pin and prosthetic replacement for the ligament of the head of the femur has been performed to stabilize the coxofemoral luxations. The surgical approach and technique for toggle pin construction used in this dog are similar to those that have been previously described; however, recent modifications have proven useful. The femoral tunnel is drilled from the lateral subtrochanteric region of the femur to the fovea capitis

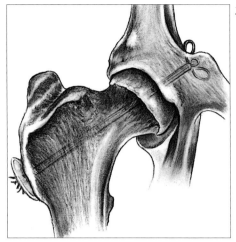

30c

by use of a C-guide. Securing the prosthetic suture through a second transverse bone in the subtrochanteric region of the femur has been abandoned. Instead, a 2-hole polypropylene button is used to tighten the suture prosthesis on the lateral aspect of the third trochanter (30c). The acetabular bone tunnel is drilled with a 3.5 mm bit and the femoral neck bone tunnel with a 2.5 mm bit. Four strands of nylon suture material (0 or 1) are used for the ligament prosthesis. Partial or complete capsulorrhaphy using polydioxanone or polyglyconate sutures may augment joint capsule healing. Although not essential to gain adequate exposure, an osteotomy of the greater trochanter was performed to approach the right coxofemoral joint. This dog's hindlimbs were not placed in coaptation after surgery and a towel sling was used to assist ambulation during the first 96 hours after surgery. It is preferable to avoid the use of non-weight-bearing slings in dogs with coxofemoral luxations and multiple limb trauma. Internal fixation and early weight-bearing is considered superior to external immobilization for treatment of many orthopedic injuries. Surgical stabilization of this dog's coxofemoral luxation with the toggle pin technique avoided bilateral external coaptation of the hindlimbs, thus minimizing the nursing care required to manage a large dog during the period of early joint capsule healing.

31 The acetabulum develops as an extension of the ossification of the three bones which form the os coxae (innominate bone): ischium, ilium and pubis. In addition, two further centers aid in its formation: the acetabular bone in the depth of the concavity and a 'T'-shaped os coxa quartum which reaches the cranial acetabular edge with its upper part and the caudal area with its lower part.

32 A bone scan of the distal hindlimbs of a young racing Greyhound with a history of running wide on the turns and performing poorly in its last three races (32a). The dog has exhibited a subtle right hindlimb lameness immediately following racing which resolves over the subsequent 24–48 hours.
i. What radiopharmaceutical is most commonly used for bone scans?
ii. What abnormality is present on the bone scan?
iii. What is the most likely diagnosis?

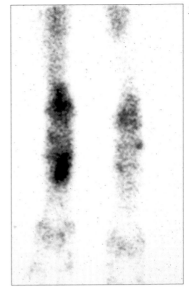

32a

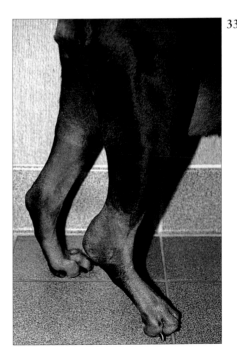

33

33 An eight-year-old, spayed female, overweight Doberman Pinscher with a four-month history of weight-bearing lameness on the right hindlimb is shown (33). When weight-bearing on the affected limb, the tibiotarsal joint is flexed, as are the metatarsophalangeal and proximal interphalangeal joints.
i. What is the diagnosis?
ii. Explain the unique postural changes present in this dog.
iii. What diagnostic procedure should be performed before formulating a treatment plan?
iv. Briefly describe recommended treatment and prognosis.

32 i. Technetium 99m-methylene diphosphonate (^{99m}TcMDP). This radiopharmaceutical is adsorbed onto the hydroxyapatite crystal of bone and there is preferential uptake in areas of increased bone metabolism. Bone phase images are typically acquired two hours following intravenous injection of the radiopharmaceutical. A vascular phase (nuclear angiogram) and soft tissue phase precede the bone phase.

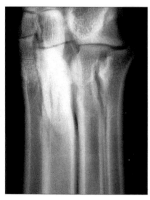
32b

ii. Focal tracer accumulation is seen at the proximal metatarsal bone of the 3rd digit. Although scintigraphy is very sensitive for detection of abnormalities in bone metabolism, scintigraphic findings are non-specific. Any cause of increased bone metabolism or remodeling (trauma, infection, neoplasia, healing fracture, degenerative joint disease) can result in focal accumulation of the radiopharmaceutical.

iii. The most likely diagnosis is a stress fracture, which was confirmed by the finding of sclerosis and an incomplete fracture of the third metatarsal on radiographs (32b). This type of fracture occurs in bones that are not able to remodel adequately in response to repeated stresses. Stress fractures are initially incomplete but can progress to complete fractures if exercise is not curtailed. Bone scintigraphy is useful for the early diagnosis of stress fractures before complete failure occurs. Bone scintigraphy can detect stress fractures before radiographic changes are apparent. Bone scintigraphy is also a valuable diagnostic modality to rule out stress fractures; a negative bone scan will reliably eliminate a stress fracture as a differential diagnosis.

33 i. Chronic injury to the Achilles or common calcaneal tendon, specifically a separation of the tendon of the gastrocnemius muscle and the common tendon of the gracilis, biceps femoris and semitendinosus muscles from the calcaneal tuber. The tendon of the superficial digital flexor muscle is still intact.

ii. Separation of the tendon of the gastrocnemius muscle and the common tendon of the gracilis, biceps femoris and semitendinosus muscles from the calcaneal tuber results in the tibiotarsal joint being held in flexion during weight-bearing. Consequently, increased tension is placed on the intact superficial digital flexor tendon during weight-bearing, resulting in flexion of the metatarsophalangeal and proximal interphalangeal joints. The unique postural changes give a 'claw' appearance to the digits.

iii. Radiographic evaluation of the crus including the stifle and tarsal joints. The position of the fabellae (origin of the gastrocnemius muscle) and appearance of the tuber calcanei (insertion of the gastrocnemius muscle and the common tendon) require special attention.

iv. The three components of the Achilles tendon are identified. The two separated tendons are sutured to the calcaneal tuber using an appropriate tendon suture pattern proximally, and a small transverse tunnel is drilled in the calcaneus to their insertions. The tibiotarsal joint is immobilized in extension during the first three weeks of the convalescence period to eliminate excessive tension on the repair.

34 A lateral view radiograph of the antebrachium of an 11-month-old, male German Shepherd Dog that presented with a history of an intermittent non-weight-bearing lameness of the left forelimb of one week's duration (34a).
i. Describe the radiographic abnormalities.
ii. What histopathologic features are characteristic of this condition?
iii. List the most common sites of occurrence of this condition.

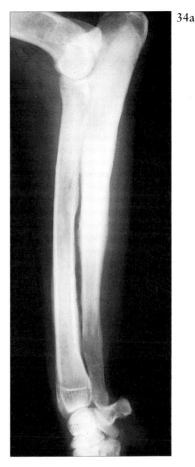

34a

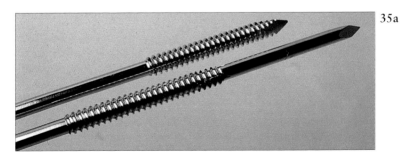

35a

35 A photograph of two external skeletal fixation pins (35a). Describe the pins.

34 i. Increased intramedullary radio-density of the proximal two-thirds of the ulna and the diaphysis of the radius, periosteal proliferation and cortical thickening of the radius and ulna, and sclerosis of the cortical bone surrounding the nutrient foramen of the radius. These changes are consistent with panosteitis. The radiographic signs of panosteitis are divided into three phases. The early phase is characterized by a granular increase in intramedullary radiodensity with loss of corticomedullary distinction. Some authors state that the early phase is preceded by a decrease in medullary radiodensity centered around the nutrient artery. The middle phase is characterized by a change in the intramedullary radiodensity to a patchy or mottled appearance. The density of the medullary canal may appear similar to that of cortical bone in this phase. These changes may be centered around the nutrient foramen. Periosteal and endosteal new bone formation resulting in cortical thickening develops during this phase. Subsequent to remodeling, the appearance of the medullary canal returns to normal, which is characteristic of the late phase. The thickened cortices and an accentuated trabecular pattern are the last to resolve.

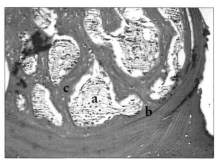

34b

ii. Panosteitis is characterized by fibroblastic and osteoblastic activity (**34b**). Initially, there is a fibroblastic response during which the normal marrow components are replaced by fibrous tissue (a). This response is centered around the nutrient artery and small medullary blood vessels. The fibrous tissue is subsequently replaced by bone through intramembranous ossification. There is concurrent cortical remodeling with periosteal, and especially endosteal (b), proliferation and short woven bone trabeculae protrude into the medullary canal. The trabeculae become thickened (c) as the condition progresses.

iii. Panosteitis occurs most commonly in the diaphysis of the proximal ulna, central radius, proximal and distal humerus, proximal and central femur, and proximal tibia. Less commonly, the metacarpal bones and pelvis may be affected.

35 i. Partially-threaded pins with a positive thread profile, one being end-threaded and the other centrally-threaded. These pins are manufactured such that the thread profile is raised above the core diameter of the pins. This design is preferable to pins with a negative thread profile in which the thread is recessed or scored into the core diameter of the pins (**35b**). The negative thread core junction acts as a stress riser which predisposes the pin to breakage and generates high strain in the bone which can result in premature fixation pin loosening.

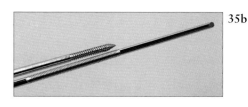

35b

36 With regard to the photograph in 35a, list two acceptable bone insertion methods for these types of fixation pins.

37 Photographs of the left forelimb of a racing Greyhound that sustained an acute forelimb injury during training, but was presented for examination three days after the injury occurred (37a, b).
i. What specific soft tissue injury is being pointed to by the examiner?
ii. What mechanical forces produce this type of injury?
iii. Muscle injuries in racing Greyhounds have been classified by Hill into three stages. Briefly define each stage as well as which injuries require surgical repair.

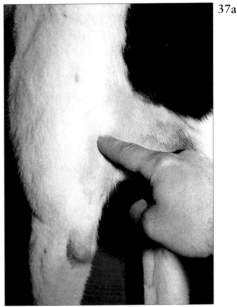

37a

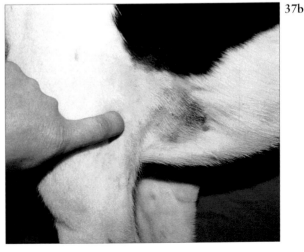

37b

36 A pre-drilling technique is the preferred method for placement of pins with positive profile threads. A twist drill bit (slightly smaller in diameter than the core diameter of the fixation pin) is used to drill pilot holes in the near and far cortices of the bone. The drilling should be performed through a small (>1 cm) incision in the skin and soft tissues. The skin is incised with a sharp scalpel while the opening through intervening soft tissues is created with a hemostat down to the bone. Prior to making the incisions, the joints proximal and distal to the bone are placed in a normal weight-bearing angle. Soft tissues can be protected from the drill with a tissue guard, but this is less necessary when adequately large openings are created. The insertion incisions result in less soft tissue trauma during fixation pin insertion and less rubbing of soft tissue on the threads of the fixation pins post-operatively, and they encourage drainage in the early post-operative period. The insertion incisions mitigate patient morbidity as a result of a healthy and comfortable fixation pin/soft tissue/bone environment. Once the pilot holes are drilled, the threaded fixation pin is inserted using either a low speed (<250 rpm) power drill or a Jacob's hand chuck.

Some surgeons consider it acceptable to insert threaded fixation pins exclusively with a slow speed (<250 rpm) power drill without pre-drilling pilot holes; however, clinical experience favors a pre-drilling technique. Insertion of fixation pins with a hand chuck without pre-drilling is unacceptable because the pin 'wobble' associated with hand chuck insertion results in bone holes larger than the diameter of the fixation pin and a loose fixation pin–bone interface. Inserting pins with a high speed drill is also unacceptable because this causes thermal necrosis of the bone, resulting in bone resorption and a loose fixation pin–bone interface.

37 i. A rupture of the long head of the triceps or so-called 'monkey' muscle. This is the most common muscular injury to the forelimb incurred by racing Greyhounds. The muscle usually avulses from its origin on the caudal surface of the scapula.
ii. Powerful active contraction of a flexor motor unit during forced passive joint extension.
iii. Stage I: myositis: simple contusion, bruising, or inflammation of a muscle.
Stage II: myositis with tearing of the muscle fascial sheath.
Stage III: tearing of the muscle fascial sheath with physical disruption of muscle fibers and hematoma formation.
Primary surgical repair is generally reserved for stage III muscle injuries but is dependent on which muscle is torn and the extent and the location of the injury. Primary surgical repair of a torn or ruptured muscle is recommended because myofibrils heal with less fibrous tissue, which leads to a more optimal return to function. Without surgical intervention, stage III muscle injuries will heal by second intention with chronic elongation of the muscle, resulting in a reduction of the functional properties of the myotendinous unit.

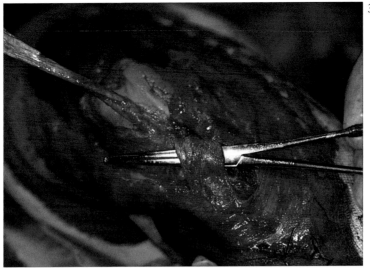

38 An intraoperative photograph of the stifle of a dog which is undergoing an intra-articular stabilization of the stifle joint for treatment of a torn CCL (38).
i. Discuss the strength and stiffness of autogenous tissues commonly used for intra-articular stabilization of CCL injuries.
ii. Discuss the concept of isometric tensioning of these grafts.

39 i. What type of bone plate is depicted (39)?
ii. Discuss the functional significance of the oval-shaped screw holes in the plate.
iii. Why is it advisable to pre-bend a straight plate in the fracture plane when the plate is applied to a flat bone surface when stabilizing a transverse fracture?

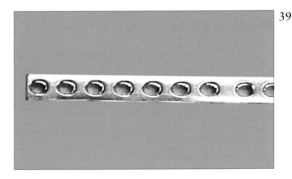

38 i. Intra-articular techniques involve placement of autogenous tissue through the joint to mimic the course of the CCL. Tissues commonly used in dogs include the medial third of the patella tendon with proximal fascia, the central third of the patella tendon and the lateral third of the patella tendon with distal fascia lata. A comparison of autografts showed a significant greater maximum load, energy absorbed and stiffness for the central third patella tendon and lateral patella tendon/distal fascia lata grafts compared with the medial patella tendon graft. Based on *in vitro* analysis, the central patella tendon graft and lateral patella tendon/distal fascia lata graft are expected to function elastically within the normal physiologic range of the CCL. However, certain mechanical and biologic factors, as discussed below, may alter the outcome.

ii. An intra-articular graft is said to be isometrically placed when the distance between points of fixation at the femur and tibia remains constant throughout flexion and extension. If there is no change in the distance between these two points of attachment, then there is no change in the length of the graft during flexion and extension. If minimal or no change in graft length occurs during passive flexion and extension, increases in strain above that initially set at graft fixation are minimal or absent since strain is equivalent to the change in length/original length. Eliminating or minimizing increases or decreases in graft stress (strain) during passive flexion/extension is beneficial in predicting joint kinematics. Excessively high graft stress would overconstrain the joint and prevent normal craniocaudal translation. This would lead to abnormal cartilage wear and/or premature stretching or rupture of the graft. Low graft stress would underconstrain the joint allowing continued instability and subsequent osteoarthritis. Isometric graft placement in the dog corresponds to a tibial tunnel placed just cranial to the medial tibial eminence and a femoral tunnel positioned at the caudodistal extent of the normal CCL's origin. Alternatively, the 'over and under' technique approaches isometric placement. Ideally, the graft should be placed 'near isometric' and secured with the stifle in normal standing position to mild extension. Tension on the graft should not exceed 1–2 kg and it is not necessary to completely eliminate all cranial drawer movement.

39 i. A dynamic compression plate often referred to as a DCP.
ii. The oval-shaped holes are designed to generate compression at the fracture/osteotomy site. An incline plane is positioned at the edge of the oval holes furthest away from the center of the plate. When a screw is positioned eccentrically in the oval hole, the head of the screw will contact the incline plane as the screw is tightened, and the plate and the bone will shift longitudinally relative to each other. The plate will be loaded in tension and the bone loaded in compression.
iii. The use of axial compression with a plate is useful in transverse fractures, providing greater stability, earlier union, and earlier weight-bearing. When a straight plate is applied to a flat bone surface, there is a region of high compressive forces beneath the plate followed by decreasing compressive forces moving away from the plate and toward the *trans*-cortex. Gapping may occur at the *trans*-cortex. Pre-bending the plate, which slightly overcontours the plate, results in application of higher compressive forces to the *trans*-cortex, eliminating the gap. *In vitro* testing has shown that pre-bending the plate increases the structural integrity and stability of the fracture repair.

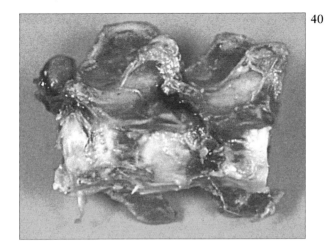

40 A photograph of two lumbar vertebrae (a vertebral motion unit) from a dog (40). The paraspinal musculature has been removed.
i. Which structure contributes the most rotational stability to the vertebral motion unit in the picture?
ii. What effect does facetectomy have on rotational stability?

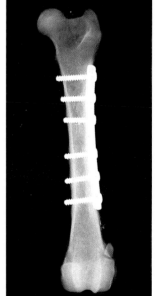

41 This is a craniocaudal view radiograph of a femur harvested from a dog (41a). A bone plate was applied to the lateral surface of the femur. A thin layer of PMMA was interposed between the bone plate and the lateral femoral cortex.
i. What is the term for the fracture fixation technique in which PMMA is placed between a bone plate and the bone?
ii. What effect does this technique have on stability of the fracture repair?
iii. What effect does this technique have on the vascularity and porosity of cortical bone?

40 i. The paired vertebral body/annulus fibrosis unit. The exact percentage of the total strength varies according to the anatomic site. The lumbar vertebral body/annulus fibrosis contributes a greater percentage of strength to that motion unit than does the vertebral body/annulus in a cervical vertebral motion unit. The rotational stability of the vertebral column can never be considered without considering the effect of the surrounding musculature in a live animal. The biomechanical values determined by bench research are only a guide to the *in vivo* dynamics of vertebral column stability. The biomechanical values may have greater significance in a paralyzed or severely traumatized animal.

ii. Unilateral facetectomy, assuming that the facet removal is complete and there is total loss of contact between the two adjacent vertebrae at that point, results in 10–20% reduction in rotational stability. Bilateral facetectomy results in the rotational stability of that vertebral motion unit being solely dependent on the paired vertebral body/annulus fibrosis unit and results in a 20–40% reduction in rotational stability. This has clinical importance in animals with vertebral body fractures. If the articular facets are intact, performing either a hemi- or a dorsal laminectomy will further destabilize the fracture, as both procedures require the removal of some or all of the articular facet. The lamina of the vertebrae form the base to which the facets are attached to the vertebral body. In this respect the lamina can be regarded as part of the biomechanical structure of the facets. Fracture or excision of the lamina that supports the facet will have the same biomechanical effect as fracture of the facet itself.

41 i. Plate luting.

ii. PMMA is placed between the plate and the cortex of the bone to increase the area of bone–plate contact. This allows transmission of load between the plate and bone by conforming to irregularities in the bone–plate interface. Studies in horses and sheep have shown that luting increases the number of cycles to failure of the bone plate and decreases the incidence of broken or loose screws. Plate luting increases the interfacial shear strength between the bone and plate, thereby protecting screws from excessive loading.

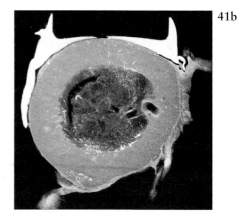

41b

iii. Dog femurs luted with PMMA had decreased vascularity to the outer one-third of the cortex and normal or increased vascularity to the inner two-thirds of the cortex five weeks after implantation. Cortical porosity was increased and the percentage of osteocyte-filled lacunae was decreased under luted plates. Ten weeks after implantation, vascularity was increased throughout the cortex under luted plates. Luting a bone plate with PMMA results in a transient loss of vascular perfusion to the outer one-third of the cortex and causes death of osteocytes in the cortical bone beneath the luted plate (**41b**).

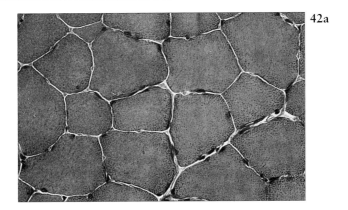

42a

42 A photomicrograph of a fresh frozen muscle biopsy sample showing normal muscle stained with H & E (**42a**).
i. Why are frozen sections essential for the morphologic evaluation of muscle biopsies?
ii. What are three clinical indicators of neuromuscular disease?
iii. What are three causes of atrophy in skeletal muscle?
iv. What is the most useful stain for distinguishing fiber types in muscle?
v. Describe the muscle fiber types present in domestic animals and correlate this with each muscle fiber types' physiologic activity.

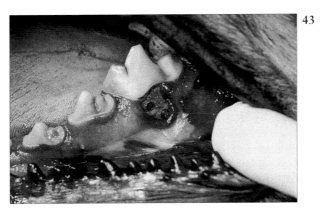

43

43 An intraoral photograph of the left mandibular first molar area taken following removal of an external skeletal fixator that was used in this dog to stabilize a mandibular fracture (**43**).
i. What complication has occurred?
ii. What is the cause of this complication?

42 i. Frozen sections minimize artifactual changes that occur with routine formalin fixation and paraffin embedding. Most importantly, there is retention of the enzymatic activity necessary for histochemical staining and determination of muscle fiber types. Evaluation of muscle fiber types is critical for the diagnosis of several neuromuscular disorders.

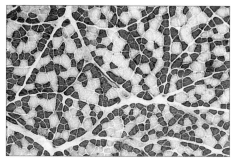
42b

ii. (1) Muscle weakness that may be generalized (e.g. paresis or paralysis, gait abnormalities or exercise intolerance) or localized (e.g. dysphagia, dysphonias, dyspnea, regurgitation). (2) Muscle atrophy or hypertrophy. (3) Muscle pain (myalgia) or stiffness.

iii. (1) Denervation atrophy as a result of neuropathies affecting motor neurons. (2) Atrophy of type 2 fibers secondary to excess GCs as a result of Cushing's syndrome or long-term corticosteroid treatment. This may result in marked muscle atrophy, particularly of the masticatory muscles, and severe muscle weakness. (3) Atrophy due to cachexia or disuse which results in a uniform decrease in size of myofibers.

iv. The myofibrillar ATPase reaction performed at an alkaline pH and following acid pre-incubation. Normally there is a checkerboard pattern of muscle fiber types as a result of innervation of myofibers by motor units (42b – ATPase reaction at pH 9.8).

v. Type 1 fibers are innervated by slow-twitch motor neurons and are light staining at an alkaline pH. Type 2 fibers are innervated by fast-twitch motor neurons and are dark staining at an alkaline pH. Type 2 fibers may be further subdivided based on the acid lability of their ATPase staining properties. Type 2A fibers (fast-twitch, fatigue resistant) and type 2B fibers (fast-twitch, fatiguable) may be identified following pre-incubations at pH 4.5 and 4.3 respectively. Two other subtypes, including type 2C fibers (developing and undifferentiated muscle) and type 2M fibers (canine masticatory muscles), are acid stable.

43 i. There is a necrotic fragment of exposed mandibular bone subjacent to the carnassial tooth which is most likely a sequestrum. There are two holes in this bone that are tracks from the fixation pins. The adjacent buccal mucosa is inflamed.

ii. This type of sequestrum is often referred to as a 'ring' sequestrum because a ring of dead bone circumscribes the fixation pin. Ring sequestra are the result of thermal injury to the bone secondary to frictional heat produced during fixation pin application. Low speed (<300 rpm) pin placement or pre-drilling of a guide hole with a twist drill bit are recommended techniques to avoid this complication. Saline lavage also helps dissipate heat during pin placement. Finally, tooth roots should be avoided during placement. Tooth root structures are harder than alveolar bone and will increase the frictional heat produced during pin placement. Tooth root injury may lead to pulpitis and eventual loss of the tooth.

44 With regard to the dog in 43, describe an appropriate treatment plan to resolve this problem.

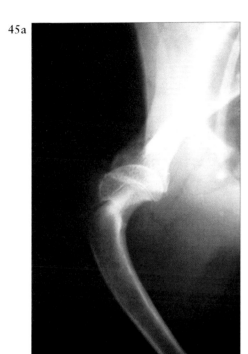

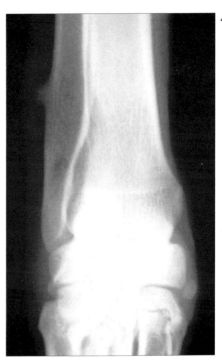

45 A lateral view radiograph of the right scapulohumeral joint of a five-month-old, female Toy Poodle with a weight-bearing lameness of the right forelimb (45a).
i. What is the diagnosis?
ii. What would be the most appropriate treatment for this dog?

46 A dorsopalmar view radiograph of the right distal antebrachium and carpus of a four-year-old Rhodesian Ridgeback, which was presented for evaluation because the owners became concerned when they had palpated a firm lump on the lateral aspect of the distal antebrachium (46).

What is the lesion affecting the distal disphyseal–metaphyseal junction of the ulna?

44 Components of the treatment plan should include sequestrectomy, extraction of the first molar, debridement of devitalized tissue, alveoloplasty, copious saline lavage and mucosal apposition over the alveolus. Soft tissue closure should be 'loose' enough to allow drainage, yet minimize access to the alveolus by foreign material and food. Feeding food of liquid or gruel consistency and lavaging of the wound after feeding during the first week following surgery should minimize wound healing complications. Antimicrobial therapy is usually not necessary if the infection is appropriately treated locally. Microbial culture of the sequestrum would likely yield a polymicrobic result indicating broad-spectrum antimicrobial therapy.

45 i. Medial luxation of the right scapulohumeral joint which is presumed to be congenital. The glenoid cavity is abnormally flat, indicating a congenital or developmental abnormality. The craniocaudal view radiograph confirmed dysplasia of the glenoid cavity.

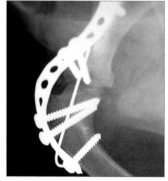

45b

ii. Closed reduction and coaptation can be sucessful if the bony conformation of the scapulohumeral joint is relatively normal. Dogs with persistent lameness and/or conformational abnormalities of the scapulohumeral joint are generally candidates for surgery. Medial transposition of the tendon of origin of the biceps brachii muscle can be used to provide medial stability if degenerative or dysplastic changes are absent or mild. In dogs with severe degenerative joint disease, severe glenoid dysplasia or failed attempts at surgical stabilization, excision arthroplasty or arthrodesis can be considered. Glenoid excision yields acceptable limb function. Two modifications of the procedure have been described, one in which the ventral angle of the scapula is excised and the second in which both the humeral head and the ventral angle of the scapula are excised. In this dog a scapulohumeral arthrodesis was performed using a veterinary cuttable plate (**45b**). A 16-month postoperative radiograph confirmed arthrodesis of the joint (**45c**). The dog had excellent limb function.

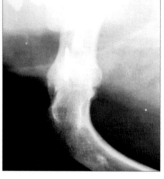

45c

Arthrodesis of the scapulohumeral joint generally yields excellent limb function with minimal alterations in gait characterized by circumduction of the limb during the swing phase of the stride.

46 An osteochondroma. Osteochondromas are benign cartilagenous capped exostoses located on the surface of bones. Osteochondromas develop in immature animals and stop growing when the animal reaches skeletal maturity. Osteochondromas can be single or multiple. Malignant transformation has been reported, but is rare.

47 A five-year-old German Shepherd Dog is presented with a left hindlimb weight-bearing lameness of seven weeks' duration. The lameness had an insidious onset, has become progressively more severe, and is characterized by a short-ened stride with a rapid, elastic internal rotation of the paw, hock and stifle, and external rotation of the tuber calcanei (arrow) during the mid-to-late swing phase of the stride (**47a**).

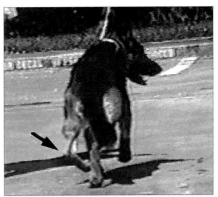
47a

i. What is the tentative diagnosis?
ii. What specific physical examination abnormalities are typically present with this condition?
iii. What is the treatment for this condition?

48 An immediate post-operative cranio-caudal view radiograph of the right tibia of a dog that has undergone a sequestrectomy and temporary stabilization with an external fixator (**48**). Antibiotic impregnanted PMMA beads have been implanted as part of the treatment for the osteomyelitis.

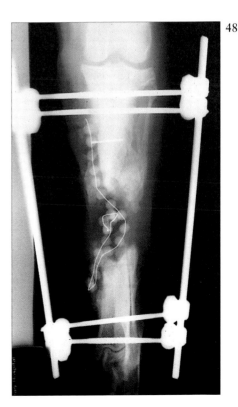
48

i. What advantages do antibiotic impregnated PMMA beads provide over systemic antibiotic therapy for treatment of osteomyelitis?
ii. What antibiotics are effectively released from PMMA beads?

47 i. This distinctive lameness is associated with myopathy of the gracilis or
semitendinosus muscles in which the
affected muscle is replaced by dense
regular connective tissue. The condition is recognized most frequently in
German and Belgian Shepherd Dogs,
and is produced by functional shortening of the affected muscle which limits
abduction of the coxofemoral joint
and extension of the stifle and hock.

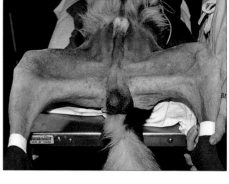

47b

ii. The distal myotendinous portion of
the affected muscle, located on the
medial aspect of the stifle, is palpably thickened and fibrotic. Definition of which
muscle is affected is determined by tracing the taut muscle band proximally to its
origin. The gracilis muscle has its origin on the pubic symphysis, while the semitendinosus muscle has its origin on the caudoventral portion of the lateral angle of the
ischiatic tuberosity. If affected dogs are positioned in dorsal recumbency, it should be
apparent that abduction of the coxofemoral joint and extension of the stifle and hock
are limited. This may be somewhat less obvious if the condition is bilateral, as in the
dog in 47b. Abduction of the coxofemoral joint or direct digital pressure on the
affected muscle may elicit a pain response.
iii. A treatment resulting in permanent resolution of lameness has not been established.
Medical treatments such as systemic or intralesional steroids, NSAIDs and acupuncture
have been ineffective. Any surgical procedure which disrupts the continuity of the
affected muscle is associated with immediate improvement in coxofemoral abduction,
increased stifle and hock extension and resolution of lameness; however, reformation of
the fibrous band and lameness has recurred two to six months following surgery in all
cases reported with adequate follow-up. Adjunctive post-surgical therapies, such as
corticosteroids, NSAIDs and lathyrogenic agents, have been ineffective in suppressing
fibroplasia and preventing the recurrence of lameness.

48 i. Advantages are associated with local release of a potent antibiotic and include: (1)
Decreased risk of toxicity. (2) Decreased risk of allergic reaction. (3) Greater local and
sustained concentration of antibiotic at the site of infection than with systemic administration. (4) Ability to treat aggressive patients (i.e. intractable animals in which the
administration of systemic antibiotic would be difficult). (5) The luxury of using an
expensive and potent antimicrobial in the beads that would otherwise be too expensive
to use systemically.
ii. Gentamicin, tobramycin, amikacin and vancomycin are the most commonly incorporated antimicrobials in PMMA beads. These drugs are all potent bactericidal, water-
soluble, heat-stable antibiotics with low tissue toxicity and good elution properties.

49 With regard to the dog in **48**, what factors affect elution of antibiotic from the PMMA beads?

50 A photograph of a histologic section through the humeral head of a ten-month-old Keeshound (**50a**). Name and describe each of the lettered structures.

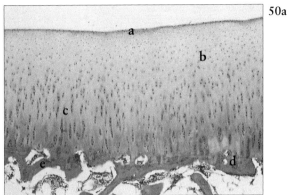

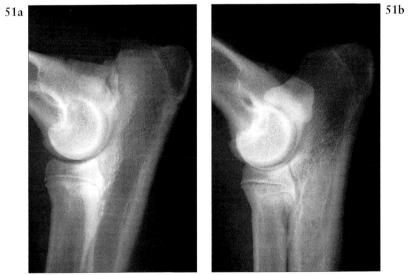

51 Lateral view radiographs of the right (**51a**) and left (**51b**) elbows of a six-and-a-half-month-old, female German Shepherd Dog. The dog presented for a left forelimb lameness which was principally ascribed to panosteitis of the left ulna. The right anconeal process has not fused with the remainder of the ulna.

At what age should the anconeal process fuse with the remainder of the ulna?

49 The surface area of the bead; type and porosity of the cement; antibiotic concentration; diffusion properties of the antibiotic; and vascularity of the surrounding tissue (i.e. fluid flow past the implant).

50 (a) The tangential or gliding zone is the most superficial layer of the articular cartilage closest to the joint surface. Chondrocytes are elongated and flattened and lie parallel to the long axis of the joint surface. Type II collagen fibers condense to form the lamina that runs along the cartilage surface in this zone.

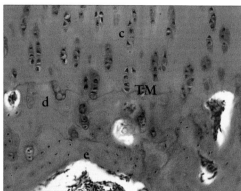

(b) The transitional zone is subjacent to the tangential zone. Chondrocytes in this zone are ovoid and randomly distributed. The hyaline cartilage matrix appears to have a random distribution of type II collagen fibers, but electron microscopy shows collagen fibers to be arranged transverse to the articular surface.

(c) The radial zone is subjacent to the transitional zone and has small chondrocytes arranged in short columns, similar to that observed in the columnar zone of the growth plate. In this zone the collagen fibers are large and tend to be oriented perpendicular to the long axis of the articular surface.

(d) The deepest region of the articular cartilage is the calcified zone. The calcified zone is characterized by small chondrocytes and a matrix that is heavily calcified. An undulating basophilic line called the tide mark (TM) separates the radial zone from the calcified zone. On higher magnification the tide mark, which is the interface between mineralized and unmineralized cartilage, is clearly visible (**50b**). Above the tide mark on the joint side, all of the cartilage receives its nutrition from the synovial fluid by diffusion. Deep to the tide mark, the mineralized cartilage is nourished by the epiphyseal vessels. Cell division may occur above the tide mark and there is migration of true articular chondrocytes toward the joint surface. Cell division may also occur below the tide mark in calcified cartilage under certain pathologic conditions; in these instances the bone may grow in minute, incremental lengths.

(e) The subchondral bone plate is a transverse plate of bone located subjacent to the calcified zone. The subchondral bone is directly continuous with the cancellous bone of the epiphysis. The bony plate and adjacent trabeculae may increase in thickness (stiffness) with various types of arthritis.

51 In most breeds of dog between 16 and 24 weeks of age.

52 A lateral view radiograph of the left humerus of a six-month-old, male Boxer that was febrile and had a non-weight-bearing lameness of the left forelimb (52). The left shoulder region was swollen and painful on manipulation. There was no evidence of an external wound. *Staphylococcus aureus* was cultured from a deep bone aspirate of the proximal humerus.
i. Describe the factors that make juvenile dogs more susceptible to hematogenous osteomyelitis than adult dogs.
ii. Briefly outline a therapeutic protocol for this dog.

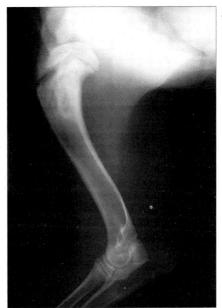

53 An immediate post-operative lateral view radiograph of the scapulohumeral joint of a five-month-old, female Dalmatian (53).
i. Describe the injury which has been repaired.
ii. The injury could not be anatomically reduced at surgery, resulting in incongruency at the articular surface of the glenoid cavity. Name the most likely long-term sequela to this incongurency and the pathophysiologic mechanisms by which this process occurs.

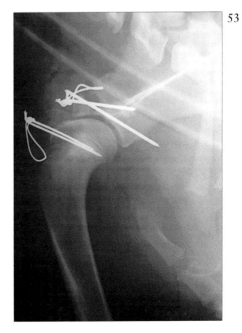

52 i. The morphology of the metaphyseal microvasculature subjacent to the growth plate predisposes this site to colonization of blood-borne organisms. Until recently, localization of bacteria in the metaphysis was attributed to sluggish blood flow in capillary loops entering large venous sinusoids. Recent studies suggest, however, that the metaphyseal capillary endothelium is discontinuous and allows extravasation of bacteria. It is in this area that bacteria, microthrombi or both lodge, resulting in avascular necrosis and an ideal environment for bacterial colonization.

ii. Aggressive antibacterial treatment and supportive care. *Staphylococcus aureus* is the most common etiologic agent and a beta-lactamase-resistant synthetic penicillin should be used pending results of aerobic and anaerobic bone aspirate or blood cultures. Supportive therapy might include analgesics to alleviate pain, fluids to maintain hydration and enteral feeding to meet caloric requirements. A lack of response to appropriate therapy within 48–72 hours may necessitate surgical intervention. The primary goal of surgery is to provide medullary decompression and drainage. Holes are drilled into the metaphysis and followed by thorough wound lavage. The incision can be closed or treated as an open wound and allowed to heal by second intention or delayed primary closure.

53 i. Avulsion fracture of the supraglenoid tuberosity of the scapula which has been repaired using a pin and tension band technique. This is most likely an avulsion fracture caused by the pull of the biceps brachii muscle which has its origin on the supraglenoid tubercle. Some investigators have suggested this lesion may be another manifestation of osteochondrosis. The second pin and tension band stabilizes the greater tubercle of the humerus which was osteotomized to facilitate exposure of the cranial region of the scapulohumeral joint. The periosteal proliferation on the cranial aspect of the scapular neck and the indistinct fracture margins suggest that the injury is chronic.

ii. Degenerative joint disease or osteoarthritis secondary to non-anatomical fracture reduction and incongruity (step defect) of the glenoid surface. Fracture non-union is also a potential complication. Osteoarthritis occurs secondary to trauma as a result of direct damage to hyaline articular cartilage at the time of injury, as well as through alterations in pressure distribution within the joint caused by articular cartilage incongruity. The degree of the articular incongruity may dictate whether osteoarthritis develops or whether the incongruity can be remodeled and joint congruity restored without significant osteoarthritis. There is evidence that small articular step defects (2 mm) can heal with fibrocartilagenous repair tissue which is continuous with the adjacent cartilage, and remodel without inciting osteoarthritis. Larger (5 mm) articular incongruities are exposed to aberrant mechanical forces that interfere with healing. The area near the articular defect is subjected to elevations in peak contact stress and increased shear stress in articular cartilage and the underlying calcified cartilage layer which causes progressive cartilage damage and degeneration. The process of cartilage degeneration involves changes in articular cartilage collagen content or loss of collagen, net loss of proteoglycans and an associated decrease in the ability of cartilage to bear and transmit forces, chondrocyte necrosis and degradation of the cartilage matrix (collagen and proteoglycans) through cytokine-mediated enzyme release or activation by chondrocytes, synoviocytes and leukocytes.

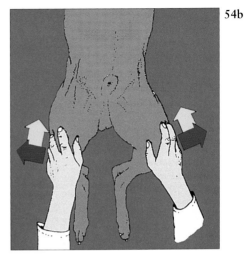

54 These two drawings illustrate an examination used to evaluate young dogs suspected of having hip dysplasia (54a, b).
i. What gait abnormalities are typically present in young dogs with hip dysplasia?
ii. What examination is being performed in the drawings?

55 These are lateral view radiographs of the distal limb of a dog diagnosed with osteosarcoma of the distal radius before (55a, left) and after (55a, right) limb-sparing surgery was performed to remove the bone tumor. The dog regained full use of the affected forelimb. What does limb-sparing surgery entail?

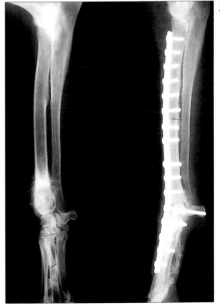

54 i. Affected dogs may have difficulty rising from a lying or sitting position. They may also exhibit lateral rotation of the pelvis by lateral bending of the lumbar spine, particularly towards the coxofemoral joint which is most painful. This minimizes the excursion of the femoral head in the acetabulum and therefore reduces the amount of pain generated in the coxofemoral joint. The dog's head may be carried lower than normal, which causes a cantilever effect and reduces the amount of weight carried by the hips. If, at the trot, the lameness is unilateral, or more pronounced in one limb, the swing phase of that limb will be reduced and slower. The stance phase will also be shortened, as the dog attempts to minimize the amount of time that the affected (or more severely affected) coxofemoral joint is loaded. In severely affected dogs there is shortening of the swing phase in the contralateral forelimb at the trot in order to accommodate the shortened swing phase of the affected hindlimb.

ii. The Ortolani examination. This examination is often performed with the dog under sedation. Although a positive Ortolani sign can be elicited in some dogs without sedation, a negative Ortolani examination can not be established unless a dog has been examined while heavily sedated or anesthetized. The dog is placed in dorsal recumbency and both femurs are positioned vertically, at right angles to the ground or table top. The stifles are flexed and axial pressure is exerted on the femurs. If laxity is present, the femoral head(s) will subluxate. The femurs are then abducted and the subluxated femoral head(s) will relocate into the acetabulum and the feeling is transmitted to the operator's hands. Relocation of the femoral head in the acetabulum may also be detectable as an audible click.

55 The marginal resection of tumor-bearing bone in patients with osteosarcoma or other primary bone neoplasms. The resected portion of bone is replaced with a cortical bone allograft, which is affixed to the host bone by standard bone plating techniques (**55b**). In some instances, such as when the scapula or distal ulna are removed, use of an allograft is not required. Limb-sparing surgery does not alter the potential for metastasis and the need for adjuvant therapy to address micrometastatic disease in patients with osteosarcoma. Currently, the most successful chemotherapeutic agent used in treatment of osteosarcoma is *cis*-diamminedichloroplatinum (*cis*-platin). Median survival times have improved from the reported four months with surgery alone to greater than ten months with surgery and *cis*-platin chemotherapy. Improvements in protocols and chemotherapeutic agents will hopefully continue to prolong survival times.

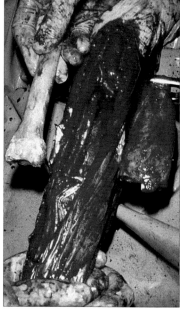

55b

56 With regard to the dog in 55:
i. What are the indications and contraindications for limb-sparing surgery in dogs?
ii. What are the benefits and disadvantages of limb-sparing surgery for dogs with osteosarcoma?

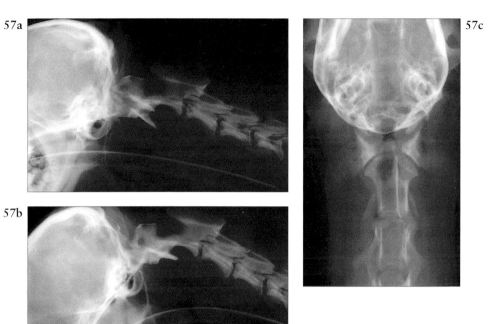

57a

57c

57b

57 Lateral (57a), flexed lateral (57b) and ventrodorsal (57c) view radiographs of the skull and cranial cervical vertebral column of a six-year-old, intact female Pekingese with an acute onset of tetraparesis.
i. Describe the radiographic abnormalities.
ii. What supporting structures must be disrupted for this condition to be present?
iii. Discuss the surgical options for treatment of this condition.

56 i. Indications are based on the need to preserve use of the limb outweighing the risk of leaving residual tumor at the surgery site. Limb sparing is a marginal and not a radical resection of cancer. The client must understand the risks as well as the benefits of this intricate procedure. Practical indications for performing limb-sparing surgery are when the dog has concurrent orthopedic or neurologic conditions that would make recovery from amputation difficult. Contraindications to performing limb-sparing surgery include when the primary tumor involves more than 50% of the length of the bone, when there is pathologic fracture or when infection or severe soft tissue inflammation is present. Each of these situations decreases the probability of a complete resection. Most dogs regain full use of the limb following limb sparing of the proximal humerus or distal radius or ulna.

ii. When performed in carefully selected cases, limb-sparing surgery maintains a functional limb for the patient and provides good quality of life without minimizing the dog's chances for survival. Complications include tumor recurrence due to inadequate excision, infection and implant or allograft failure. Tumor recurrence is the most serious of these complications and the client must be aware of the risk to their pet. Infection is the most common complication. Dogs that develop infection usually must be maintained on antibiotics for prolonged periods of time.

57 i. Atlantoaxial subluxation. There is separation of the dorsal spinous process of the axis (C2) from the dorsal arch of the atlas (C1). The dens is intact and has normal conformation. This is unusual since hypoplasia or agenesis of the dens is present in most dogs with atlantoaxial subluxation.

ii. The dens is supported by a series of ligaments. The transverse ligament firmly attaches the dens to the ventral arch of the atlas, the apical ligament attaches the apex of the dens to the ventral aspect of the foramen magnum and the paired alar ligaments attach the cranial aspect of the dens to the occipital condyles. In addition, the dorsal atlantoaxial ligament passes between the dorsal spinous process of the axis and dorsal arch of the atlas. All of these structures were probably disrupted in this case.

iii. Dorsal stabilization techniques attempt to reconstruct the torn dorsal atlantoaxial ligament through the use of a wire or non-absorbable suture prosthesis. The prosthetic ligament is passed under the dorsal arch of the atlas and secured through drill holes placed in the dorsal spinous process of the axis. The nuchal ligament can also be passed under the dorsal arch of the atlas and fixed in a notch created in the dorsal spinous process. Hemilaminectomy is usually not performed concurrently with these techniques. Ventral stabilization procedures involve either pinning or lag screw fixation of the atlantoaxial articulation. The articular cartilage is debrided with either a bone curette or a pneumatic drill and a cancellous bone graft is implanted. With the luxation reduced, either Kirschner wires or 1.5 mm cortical bone screws are placed across the articulation using the alar notch as the reference point. Ventral application of straight or T-shaped miniplates has also been reported. Surgical success rates are variable, ranging from 47% with the ventral pinning technique, 52% with the double dorsal wire, 63% with dorsal suture and 91% with ventral lag screw fixation.

58 A lateral view stress radiograph of the carpus of an eight-year-old, neutered female Schnauzer with an acute, right forelimb lameness (58a).
i. Describe the injury.
ii. What are likely sequelae of managing this injury by application of external coaptation?
iii. Describe appropriate surgical treatment of this type of injury.

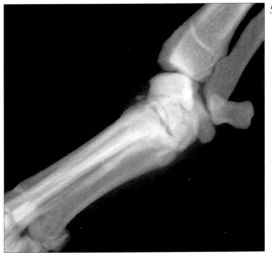

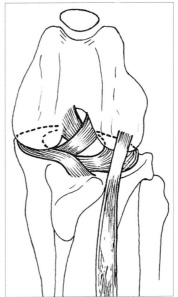

59 Drawings of the stifle of a dog in extension (59a) and flexion (59b).
i. What are the three functions of the CCL?
ii. What is the origin and insertion of the CCL?

63

58 i. This radiograph demonstrates chip fractures dorsal to the distal row of carpal bones and a severe hyperextension sprain injury with subluxation of the middle carpal and carpometacarpal joints. This implies that the palmar carpal ligaments and fibrocartilage are torn.

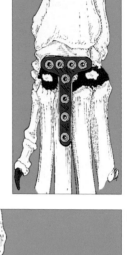

58b

ii. Healing of torn palmar carpal ligaments and fibrocartilage occurs by fibroplasia, but typically these structures regain tensile strength relatively slowly. Even following eight to twelve weeks of external coaptation, recurrence of hyperextension and carpal subluxation is usual. This is thought to be due to failure of the injured ligamentous structures to regain adequate strength. The long-term sequela is chronic osteoarthritis of the affected joints.

iii. Partial carpal arthrodesis of the middle carpal and carpometacarpal joints was performed in this dog. Partial carpal arthrodesis is preferable to pancarpal arthrodesis because it preserves motion in the antebrachiocarpal joint. A dorsal surgical approach is made to the carpus and articular cartilage of the middle carpal, carpometacarpal and intercarpal joints is debrided. Autogenous cancellous bone graft is packed into the debrided joint spaces. The two methods for internal fixation of partial carpal arthrodesis are plate fixation (58b) and use of small diameter intramedullary pins or Kirschner wires in the third and fourth metacarpal bones that are seated into the radial or ulnar carpal bones (58c). The latter technique is associated with better functional results. Following surgery, coaptation is applied to the limb to protect the internal fixation until bone union has occurred. A thick padded bandage is applied immediately after surgery until swelling subsides. This is replaced with a thinner bandage reinforced with a fiberglass splint for six to ten weeks.

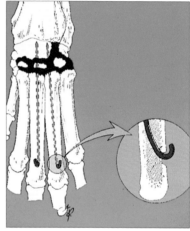

58c

59 i. (1) To prevent internal rotation of the tibia on the femur. (2) To prevent excessive cranial movement of the tibia in respect to the femur (also known as cranial drawer motion). (3) To prevent hyperextension of the stifle.

ii. The CCL originates on the caudomedial portion of the lateral femoral condyle, then transverses diagonally through the intercondylar fossa of the femur to attach on the craniomedial intercondylar area of the tibia.

60 A mass is placed onto an articular cartilage specimen and displacement is measured over a 20-second interval. The curve represents the data recorded (**60a**).

i. What is the term that describes the non-linear response shown?

ii. Why does cartilage have this property?

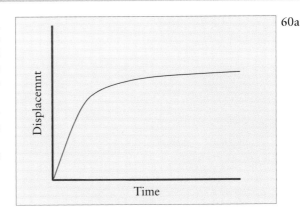

60a

61 A photograph of a five-month-old Labrador Retriever that sustained multiple fractures of the maxilla when the dog was hit by a car (**61a**). Note how the dog's maxilla deviates to the right. The dog was photographed following surgical reduction and stabilization of the maxilla with an external fixator (**61b**). An acrylic connecting column was used to construct the external skeletal fixation frame.

What diameter acrylic column has comparable mechanical characteristics to a medium Kirschner–Ehmer connecting system?

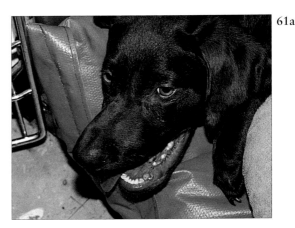

61a

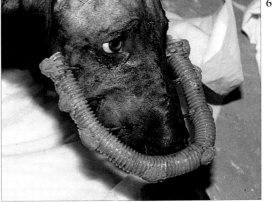

61b

60b

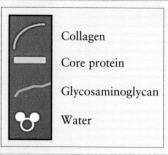

Collagen

Core protein

Glycosaminoglycan

Water

60c

60 i. Viscoelastic behavior. An important property of viscoelastic materials is that their mechanical response will vary depending on the rate at which a load is applied. If load is applied rapidly, there is less time to respond and the structure is stiffer. **ii.** Cartilage is viscoelastic because of the manner in which water is trapped in the proteoglycan molecules of the matrix. Large proteoglycan molecules are held within the organized collagen structure. Proteoglycans consist of a core protein with many attached glycosaminoglycans, the common glycosaminoglycans being chondroitin and keratin sulfates. The polyanionic nature of the chondroitin and keratin sulfate results in these molecules having a strong electronegative charge. The negatively charged glycosaminoglycans repel each other and attract and imbibe water molecules into the spaces between glycosaminoglycan subunits (60b). The density of the proteoglycan molecules is such that they are confined by the collagenous matrix and not allowed to fully hydrate. This results in a resting tissue pressure within cartilage.

When a load is applied to cartilage, the increase in pressure squeezes water out of the proteoglycan molecules (60c). As water is squeezed out of the cartilage matrix, the cartilage becomes less compliant. Movement of water requires time, thus the response of the cartilage to the load requires time.

61 An acrylic column approximately 2 cm in diameter has comparable, if not superior, mechanical properties to the medium Kirschner–Ehmer connecting system.

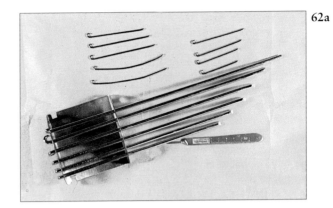

62a

62 A photograph of a specific type of orthopedic implant system (62a).
i. Name the implants.
ii. What type of fractures are best suited for this type of fixation?
iii. Are these devices frequently used in small animal orthopedics?

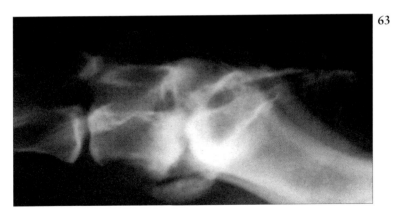

63

63 A lateral view radiograph of the lumbar vertebral column of a large, male, mixed-breed dog with lumbosacral discospondylitis (63). What radiographic criteria differentiate discospondylitis from spondylosis deformans and neoplasia of the vertebrae?

62 i. Rush pins. One end of a Rush pin is beveled and the opposite end has a hook. Properly inserted, Rush pins produce dynamic fixation. Rush pins are inserted at an acute angle to the long axis of the bone so the beveled end of each pin deflects off the endosteal cortical surface and continues up the medullary cavity. The bending of the pins created during insertion places the pins under constant tension, thus producing dynamic fixation which resists loosening. Rush pins are very effective in neutralizing bending and rotational forces.
ii. Fractures located near the ends of long bones, for example metaphyseal and physeal fractures. If Rush pins are used to stabilize physeal fractures, closure of the physis will likely occur, especially if the pins are not removed by one month following surgery.

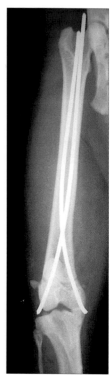

62b

iii. Rush pins are used infrequently in dogs and cats for several reasons. Inventory of a large number of pins is necessary in order to have the correct diameter and length pins available. Rush pins were designed for use in humans and appropriate diameters/lengths may not be available for smaller dogs and cats. Proper application of Rush pins is technically demanding. Pin placement requires pre-drilling a pilot hole in the smaller fracture segment with an awl. The hooked end of the pin is then engaged with an impactor to drive and seat the pin. The pins must cross after extending beyond the fracture for maximal mechanical advantage. If the pins cross at the fracture site, distraction of the fracture will occur as the pins are advanced.

The biomechanical principles of Rush pinning are commonly adapted for use in dogs and cats using small diameter Steinmann pins or Kirschner wires in 'the manner of Rush pins' (62b). The principles of dynamic fixation of Rush pinning can be achieved by inserting small diameter, and thus flexible, Steinmann pins or Kirschner wires at an acute angle to the long axis of a long bone. Chisel-point tip pins or wires should be used so that the pins or wires will deflect off, rather than penetrate, the endosteal corticies.

63　Discospondylitis is defined as infection of an intervertebral disc with concurrent osteomyelitis of the contiguous vertebrae. The most common radiographic signs associated with discospondylitis include bony lysis of one or both vertebral body end-plates and the affected vertebral bodies, bone proliferation on and within infected vertebrae, and ventral osseous proliferation bridging the disc space to varying degrees. The presence of lysis of the vertebral body and involvement of the disc space itself are key elements in differentiating this disease from benign spondylosis deformans. Neoplastic disease tends to localize within the vertebrae itself and not involve or cross the disc space.

64 With regard to the dog in **63**:
i. List three possible methods of identifying the causative organism.
ii. What organisms are most commonly associated with discospondylitis?
iii. Assuming the causative infectious agent has been identified, how long should treatment continue?

65a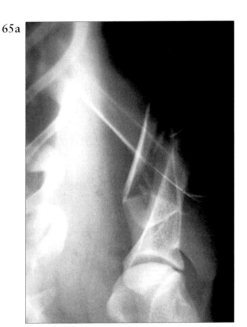

65b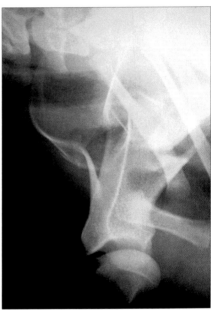

65 Craniocaudal (**65a**) and lateral (**65b**) view radiographs of the scapulohumeral region of a dog that was hit by a car and presented with a non-weight-bearing lameness of the right forelimb. Pain and swelling were localized to the right shoulder region.
i. Describe the injury.
ii. What factors influence whether conservative or surgical treatment should be employed for this type of injury?
iii. What type of fixation should be used if surgery is done?

64 i. The causative infectious agent may be identified via blood culture, urine culture, fluoroscopically-guided aspiration of the affected disc space or culture of affected bone obtained during exploratory surgery of the area. Organisms isolated from urine and blood can only be presumed as the probable cause of discospondylitis.

ii. Hematogenous discospondylitis (as opposed to that which might occur post-operatively or due to a migrating foreign body) may be either bacterial or fungal. Coagulase positive *Staphylococcus* spp. (*aureus* and *intermedius*), *Streptococcus* spp. and *Brucella canis* are most commonly isolated. Other reported bacterial causes include *Escherichia coli*, *Corynebacterium* spp. and *Proteus*. *Aspergillus* spp. is the most common fungal organism reported to cause discospondylitis and is most frequently associated with discospondylitis in German Shepherd Dogs.

iii. Dogs that do not have improvement of clinical signs within five days of the onset of antibiotic treatment should be reassessed. For dogs that show improvement and become asymptomatic, it is important to continue antibiotic treatment until resolution is documented radiographically. Radiographs should be repeated every four to six weeks until vertebral fusion has occurred or all evidence of bony lysis has resolved. Premature discontinuation of treatment often results in relapse.

65 i. There is a highly comminuted fracture of the body and spine of the right scapula.

ii. Most fractures of the body of the scapula can be treated conservatively with application of a Velpeau sling or spica splint and/or cage confinement. Three to four weeks of coaptation are generally sufficient to allow clinical union to occur. Contracture of the triceps muscles can occur as a sequela to prolonged coaptation. Open reduction and internal fixation should be considered with highly comminuted fractures or fractures inducing malposition of the glenoid cavity.

iii. Although pins and wires have been advocated for stabilization of scapular body fractures, bone plates are preferred. The plate should be applied in the angle located at the base of the spine of the scapula (**65c**). Use of a semitubular plate, applied in an inverted manner, to improve contact between the plate and the bone has been described. Veterinary cuttable plates can also be used to increase the number

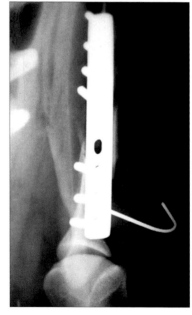

65c

of screws which can be placed in the scapula. A second plate can also be placed on the scapular spine to improve stability in selected fractures.

66a

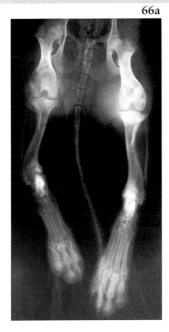

66b

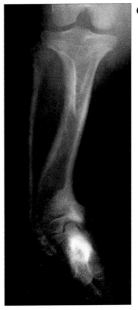

66 A nine-month-old, female Dachshund was presented with a weight-bearing lameness of the right hindlimb that the owner first noted when the dog was five months of age. There was no history of trauma. Physical examination revealed medial angulation of the distal portion of the right hindlimb. A craniocaudal view radiograph of both hindlimbs is shown (66a). An isolated craniocaudal view radiograph of the right tibia and pes is also shown (66b).

i. Describe the radiographic abnormalities.

ii. What is the diagnosis and what is the underlying pathogenesis of this syndrome?

iii. Describe the surgical procedure for correcting this dog's limb deformity.

67 A drawing illustrating a suture pattern used to perform a tenorrhaphy (67).

i. What suture pattern is illustrated?

ii. What advantages and disadvantages does this pattern have over single and double locking-loop sutures?

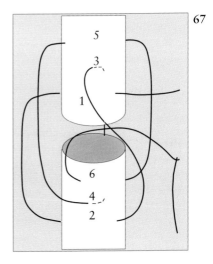

67

66 i. There is a varus deviation of the right distal tibia and pes. Although the left hindlimb has as similar but much less severe deformity, the deformity in the right hindlimb is particularly evident when the right hindlimb is compared with the left hindlimb.

ii. Pes varus (or metaphyseal dysplasia) is a condition described in juvenile Dachshunds. Premature closure of the medial aspect of the distal tibial physis retards medial tibial growth and produces a varus curvature of the bone at the medial surface of the distal metaphysis. Rotational deformity of the distal tibia can also be present.

iii. By using the contralateral limb as a template for the correction and calculating the degree of correction required geometrically, an open wedge

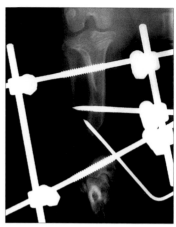

66c

osteotomy can be planned and performed. It is preferable to stabilize the osteotomy with an external fixation as was done in this case (66c). The external fixator affords the surgeon considerable latitude in adjusting the alignment of corrective osteotomy both during and following surgery while providing sufficient stability of the small distal segment. Small mini 'T'-plates and screws have also been used successfully to stabilize corrective osteotomies in the treatment of pes varus.

67 i. A triple-loop pulley pattern. The first and second bites make a near-far suture. The third and fourth bites are taken at 120° to the first suture and are of equal sizes. The final two bites are taken at 120° to the second suture and are placed to create a far-near suture. Thus, a cross-section of the repaired tendon would reveal that the loops are placed at 120° to each other.

ii. The time taken to place a single locking-loop suture is generally slightly shorter than placing a triple-loop pulley suture. Double locking-loop and triple-loop pulley sutures take a comparable time to create. Triple-loop pulley sutures had a greater resistance to gap formation than either of the locking-loop sutures and had a different mode of failure when they were compared in a model using superficial flexor tendons from fresh equine cadavers. The locking-loop sutures both failed by suture breakage but the triple-loop pulley failed first by suture pull-out and then by suture breakage.

The longitudinal sutures of the triple-loop pulley pattern are placed on the outside of the tendon, whereas in both locking-loop patterns the longitudinal sutures are within the substance of the tendon. Theoretically, placement of the logitudinal sutures outside of the tendon should cause minimal disruption of the tendon structure. A potential disadvantage of the longitudinal sutures of the triple-loop pully pattern is that the sutures may stimulate peritendinous inflammation and increase adhesion formation. In human patients this can have serious consequences since gliding function is critical. In dogs and cats, gliding function is less important and adhesion formation does not cause clinically detectable problems.

68 Schematic drawing of a segment of cortical bone (68). Identify the elements of the microstructure of bone labeled a–e.

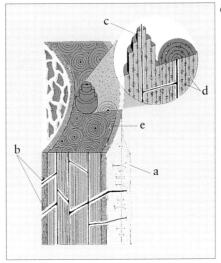

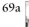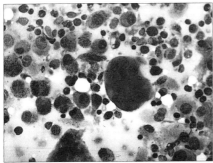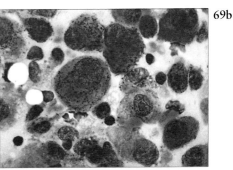

69 A nine-year-old, intact male Irish Setter was presented with an acute onset of a right forelimb lameness. Radiographically there was a pathologic fracture involving the distal metaphysis of the right radius. Bone lysis was present at the fracture site. A fine-needle aspirate of the lesion was performed and the material retrieved was evaluated cytologically (69a, b).
i. Give a cytologic description.
ii. What is the diagnosis?

68 Bone tissue is a specialized connective tissue that is made up of organic and inorganic portions that allows bone to act in a supportive capacity and as a mineral reservoir. The inorganic component gives bone its rigidity, while the organic portion makes the bone flexible. Macroscopically, all bones are composed of two types of osseous tissue: cortical bone, which forms the outer shell, and cancellous bone which is confined within the cortical bone shell. All bones are surrounded by a dense fibrous membrane, the *periosteum* (a). The outer periosteal layer is permeated by blood vessels and nerve fibers that pass into the cortex via *Volkmann's canals* (b), connecting with the *Haversian canals* (c) and extending to the cancellous bone. The inner cambium layer of the periosteum contains cells that are responsible for generating new bone during growth and repair. The periosteum covers the entire bone except at the joint surfaces, which are covered with articular cartilage. At the microscopic level, the fundamental structural unit of bone is the osteon, or Haversian system. At the center of each osteon is a small channel (Haversian canal) that contains blood vessels and nerve fibers. The osteon itself consists of a concentric series of layers, or *lamellae* (d), of mineralized matrix surrounding the central canal. Along the boundaries of each layer are cavities (lacunae) that contain a single bone cell (osteocyte). Many small channels (canaliculi) radiate from each lacuna, connecting adjacent lacunae and, ultimately, communicating with the central Haversian canal. At the periphery of each osteon is a *cement line* (e), a narrow area of cement-like ground substance composed primarily of glycosaminoglycans. Canaliculi do not cross cement lines. A typical osteon is approximately 200 microns in diameter. Most of the osteons in long bones are oriented parallel to the long axis of the bone, although osteons frequently branch and connect with other osteons.

69 i. The material is very cellular containing a predominant population of individually arranged, round-to-oval cells with low numbers of large, multinucleated giant cells. A dense, amorphous, pink material consistent with osteoid is seen extracellularly (**69a**). The majority of the cells contain variable amounts of moderately basophilic cytoplasm which often contains a granular, eosinophilic material (**69b**). Nuclei are usually eccentrically located within the cytoplasm. Many nuclei exhibit anaplastic features of malignancy such as anisokaryosis, clumped chromatin, multiple and prominent nucleoli and variable nuclear to cytoplasmic ratio. Inflammatory cells are not observed.
ii. The major considerations for possible etiologies of a pathologic fracture with evidence of bone lysis are infection, inflammation and neoplasia. The lack of neutrophils and/or macrophages in the cytologic preparation makes inflammation or infection unlikely etiologies. The presence of a monomorphic population of cells is indicative of neoplasia. The anaplastic nuclear features are typical of a malignancy and the individual arrangement of the cells is most suggestive of a sarcoma. Several types of sarcoma may involve the appendicular skeleton including osteosarcoma, fibrosarcoma, chondrosarcoma, hemangiosarcoma or giant cell sarcoma. The cytologic features of round to oval cells with eccentrically located nuclei (reminiscent of osteoblasts), multinucleated giant cells and the presence of extracellular pink material and intracytoplasmic granules consistent with osteoid, substantiate a tentative diagnosis of osteosarcoma.

70 Dogs may develop atrophy and/or swelling of the masticatory muscles which may be associated with pain on opening the jaw, inability to open the jaws and exophthalmos or enophthalmos. This is a photograph of a dog with marked temporalis muscle atrophy (70a).

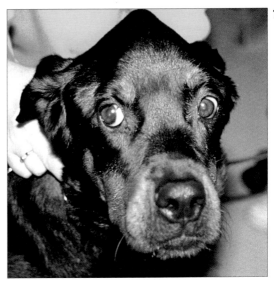

i. What is the differential diagnosis for the dog in this photograph?
ii. What anatomic and biochemical differences in the masticatory muscles could explain 'focal' muscle involvement in masticatory muscle myositis?
iii. What diagnostics should be performed in this case?
iv. What is the recommended treatment protocol for masticatory muscle myositis?

71 The proximal femur from a dog (71).
i. What anatomic structure is centered in the oval?
ii. What muscle inserts at this protuberance?

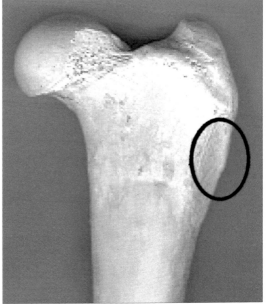

70 i. Inflammatory myopathies (masticatory muscle myositis and polymyositis); neurogenic atrophy; chronic corticosteroid therapy; retrobulbar abscess (particularly if exophthalmus present); temporomandibular joint disease.

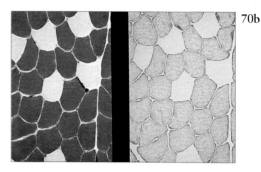

70b

ii. The masticatory muscles are innervated by the mandibular branch of the trigeminal nerve (cranial nerve V) and include the temporalis, masseter, medial and lateral pterygoideus, tensor tympani and tensor veli palatini muscles. These muscles contain unique fiber types (type 2M fibers and a variant of type 1 fibers) not found in other muscle groups.

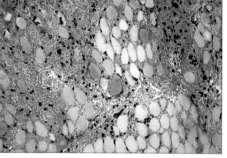

70c

iii. Should include evaluation of serum creatine kinase, immunocytochemical assay for antibodies against masticatory muscle type 2M fibers, radiographic evaluation of temporomandibular joints and a biopsy from a masticatory muscle. The muscle biopsy is essential for diagnosis and prognosis by evaluating the severity of inflammation and amount of fibrosis. A section from normal dog temporalis muscle reacted for ATPase activity (type 1 fibers stain light and type 2M fibers stain dark) (70b, left) and a serial section incubated with serum from a suspected case of masticatory muscle myositis followed by incubation with staphylococcal protein A–horseradish peroxidase (70b, right) are shown. Labeling of type 2M fibers (goldish-brown stain) is indicative of the presence of autoantibodies against this muscle fiber type. The muscle biopsy (70c) is reacted with acid phosphatase–peroxidase and demonstrates the presence of infiltrating lymphocytes (blue), macrophages (red) and eosinophils (brown).
iv. Immunosuppressive dosages of corticosteroids should be used until serum creatine kinase returns to the normal range and jaw function is regained. Dosage should then be decreased until the lowest alternate day dosage that keeps the dog free of clinical signs is obtained. This treatment regimen should be continued for four to six months. If treatment is stopped too soon, clinical signs will return. Occasionally, other immunosuppressive agents (e.g. Imuran) need to be added.

71 i. The third trochanter of the femur.
ii. The superficial gluteal muscle inserts on the third trochanter.

72 An immediate post-operative ventrodorsal view radiograph of the pelvis of an eight-month-old mixed breed dog that had an unilateral triple pelvic osteotomy (72).
i. What is the most common reason for performing a triple pelvic osteotomy?
ii. What are contraindications for performing a triple pelvic osteotomy?
iii. How is the angle of acetabular rotation determined?

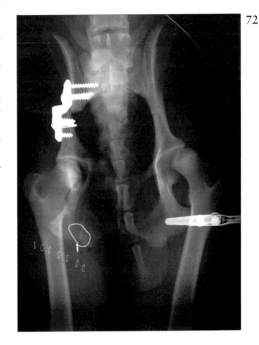

73 A cadaver specimen showing the placement of an ischio-ilial pin (DeVita pin) for stabilization of the coxofemoral joint after reduction of a craniodorsal luxation (73a, b).
i. Describe the technique for properly inserting and positioning an ischio-ilial pin.
ii. List potential complications associated with the use of ischio-ilial pins.

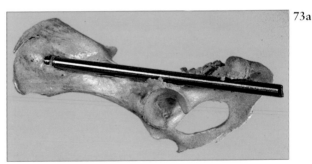

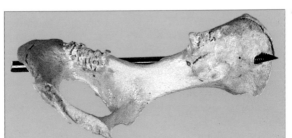

72 i. Triple pelvic osteotomy is generally performed in dogs with hip dysplasia that are less than one year of age. Best results are achieved if the surgery is done at a young age while the coxofemoral joint is developing. The purpose of performing a triple pelvic osteotomy is to prevent coxofemoral joint subluxation during weight-bearing. During surgery the acetabular segment is rotated ventrolaterally to improve acetabular coverage of the femoral head. Traumatic coxofemoral joint luxation is another less common indication.

ii. Triple pelvic osteotomies are not advocated for dogs with obvious radiographic evidence of degenerative joint disease. If there is insufficient joint surface available to achieve proper congruency, eburnation of cartilage and loss of the dorsolateral acetabular rim, the value of performing a triple pelvic osteotomy is questionable. Osteophytes on the femoral neck and dorsal acetabular rim may cause impingement and interfere with the range of motion of the coxofemoral joint, which can cause pain and decrease the benefits derived from the surgery.

iii. The angle of reduction (Ortolani sign) and the angle of subluxation (Barlow's sign) are measured. The angle of reduction is the maximum angle the acetabulum needs to be rotated in order to achieve stability. The angle of subluxation represents the minimal required angle of acetabular rotation. These two angles are used to select the appropriate implant for axial rotation of the acetabular segment. Slocum pelvic osteotomy plates are the most common implants used for stabilizing pelvic osteotomies. These plates have predetermined angles (20°, 30° and 40°) of rotation. In order to prevent overrotation of the pelvis and avoid impingement of the dorsal acetabular rim on the femoral neck, the angle of the plate selected should be closer to the angle of subluxation than to the angle of reduction.

73 i. The luxation is reduced under general anesthesia and the pin should course ventral to the ischium and pass adjacent to the dorsal acetabular rim, and the tip of the pin should be seated into the wing of the ilium. The pin is inserted ventral to the ischium through a stab incision in the skin. A palpable notch located medial and adjacent to the lateral eminence of the ischiatic tuberosity defines the proper position for insertion. This position has been shown to decrease the rate of reluxation compared to a more laterally placed pin. If the pin is inserted too medial, proper seating the tip of the pin into the ilial wing is difficult. The pin is advanced cranially over the dorsal acetabular rim and femoral head and embedded in the wing of the ilium. The use of an end-threaded pin which can be screwed in the ilium improves pin stability and decreases the incidence of pin migration. The surgeon must be aware that the pin often contacts the sciatic nerve and if an end-threaded pin is used, the pin should not be rotated until the threaded portion of the pin has been advanced cranial to the coxofemoral joint. The pin is cut below the skin surface to prevent contamination, seroma formation and trauma to the skin. The ischio-ilial pin remains in place for three to six weeks. The pin in the specimen pictured here was left as a permanent implant, inducing osteophyte formation.

ii. Complications include pin migration, reluxation, injury to the femoral head, sciatic nerve injury during pin placement, septic arthritis, pressure sores and development of draining sinus tracts. The overall success rate with ischio-ilial pinning of selected coxofemoral luxations has been reported to be 73%; the complication rate was 32%.

74 A lateral view radiograph of a dog's antebrachium which is undergoing correction of an antebrachial limb deformity and limb lengthening utilizing the Ilizarov method (74).
i. What scientific term is used to describe this phenomenon of bone lengthening?
ii. What is latency?
iii. Define the terms rate and rhythm.

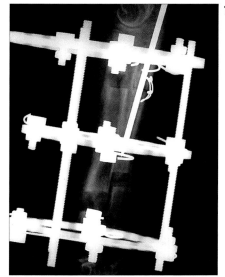

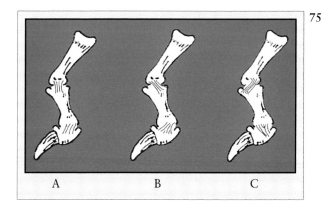

75 Phalangeal joint luxations are very common injuries in racing Greyhounds. Three possible anatomic configurations for the P1-P2 and P2-P3 collateral ligaments are represented (75).
i. Which representation is correct?
ii. Should the stability of interphalangeal ligaments be evaluated in flexion, in extension or in a neutral position?
iii. Primary surgical repair of P1-P2 and P2-P3 collateral ligaments offer the best prognosis for return to racing. List three techniques described to repair P1-P2 collateral ligaments.

74 i. Distraction osteogenesis – the formation of new bone in an osteotomy gap which is generated when stabilized bone segments undergo gradual, controlled separation. Early callus subjected to slow controlled traction is metabolically stimulated and will, under appropriate conditions, differentiate and proliferate to form bone in the distraction zone. The new bone formed under these circumstances is referred to as regenerate bone. Fixator stability, adequate blood supply, minimal disruption of periosteal soft tissues, proper rate and rhythm of distraction, and physiological use of the limb are critical to regenerate bone formation.

ii. Latency is the period of time elapsed following osteotomy before distraction is initiated. Latency is recommended to allow the initial phase of bone union to occur; this is postulated to improve osteogenesis by enhancing local cellular and vascular responses, including the formation of a fibrovascular bridge which serves as a framework for intramembranous ossification under proper conditions of stability, controlled distraction and weight-bearing. The latency period should be determined in each individual case based on the age of the animal, the bone involved, the type and location of the osteotomy and the degree of associated soft tissue trauma. Recent clinical reports suggest a three-to-five-day latency is adequate for skeletally mature dogs and cats and a one-to-three-day latency is adequate in skeletally immature dogs and cats.

iii. Rate of distraction refers to the total amount of distraction performed in a 24-hour period. Rhythm refers to the number of distraction increments per 24-hour period. Ilizarov recommended a distraction rate of 1 mm per day divided in four equal increments (0.25 mm every six hours) as the most practical rate and rhythm for producing quality regenerate bone with minimal morbidity. Rates of 0.5–2.0 mm per day have produced acceptable osteogenesis in dogs. Similarly, the rhythm can be altered to two or three increments per day, especially for bone lengthenings of 15% or less. Sporadic distraction rhythms, even at acceptable rates, disrupt the osteogenic process in the developing regenerate and should be avoided.

75 i. B. The P1-P2 collateral ligaments are directed from the dorsal aspect of the P1 to the proximal palmar aspect of the P2. The P2-P3 collateral ligaments run from the distal end of the P2 and fan out to a diffuse attachment on the P3.

ii. In extension. Testing the stability of the interphalangeal ligaments while the joint is in flexion or in neutral position can produce a false impression of laxity.

iii. Interphalangeal collateral instability can be stabilized with three or four horizontal mattress sutures placed in the torn ligament and joint capsule, followed by a single encircling purse string or Connell suture. Good results have been reported placing two or three sutures of 4-0 polydioxanone or polyglyconate in a pulley pattern through the damaged collateral ligament. Additional sutures can improve stability. The sutures must be placed in the correct anatomic alignment. Incorrect placement and overtightening of sutures are the most common technical causes of failure. Another technique is to use an autogenous tissue graft placed and sutured over the ligament with 4-0 polydioxanone. Donor sites can be the tendon of the dewclaw or a fascial graft taken from the epaxial muscles of the tail.

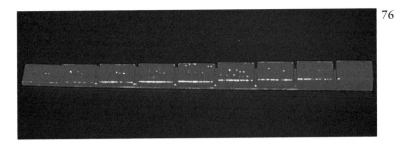

76 A photograph of a surgical implant (76).
i. What operation is performed using this orthopedic implant?
ii. What are the indications for this procedure?
iii. How is this operation performed?

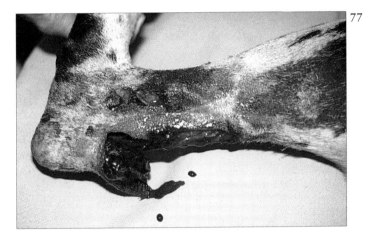

77 A photograph of the hindlimb of a two-year-old, female Great Dane that sustained an acute, traumatic laceration of the Achilles (the common calcaneal) tendon (77).
Should this injury be managed conservatively and allowed to heal by second intention or should primary tenorrhaphy be attempted?

76 i. Femoral neck lengthening. Slocum femoral neck lengthening wedges are manufactured from a polyacetyl resin. The wedges are available in left and right configurations and the segments increase in thickness from 4 mm to 12 mm. The wedges are also slightly increased in width in the proximal/distal plane.

ii. Some dysplastic dogs have an abnormally short femoral neck. Short femoral necks are common in some breeds of dogs, including Chow Chows, Akitas, and Tibetan Mastiffs. Biomechanically, the femoral neck determines the distance from the center of the femoral head to the greater trochanter. This distance creates a lever arm that directs the femoral head into the acetabulum. Femoral neck lengthening is advocated in young dysplastic dogs with either: adequate dorsal acetabular cover of the femoral head, yet insufficient medially directed resultant forces to prevent the femoral head from subluxating; or combined acetabular and femoral neck abnormalities. In the latter cases, combining femoral neck lengthening with triple pelvic osteotomy is advisable.

iii. Triple pelvic osteotomy, if indicated, is performed. The approach is extended distally to expose the lateral aspect of the femur. The biceps femoris muscle is divided from the tensor fascia lata to expose the vastus lateralis muscle. A myotenotomy of the origin of the vastus muscle group is done and the vastus muscles are reflected exposing the proximal femur and the femoral diaphysis. The cranial aspect of the femur is visualized by externally rotating the femur. Osteotomy of the femur is performed in the sagittal plane starting at the mid-point between the femoral head and the greater trochanter using a pneumatic reciprocating saw. The osteotomy is continued distally, taking care to maintain an exact sagittal plane. If wedges 8 mm or less are to be used, a 10 cm osteotomy is performed. A 15 cm osteotomy is required if wedges 9 mm or greater are needed. The osteotomy is spread open at its proximal aspect, and the appropriate size wedge is placed within the osteotomy at the level of the lesser trochanter. The femur is tested for lateral translation and, if stable, the wedge is held in place with a transcortical pin. A second wedge is placed more distal in the osteotomy and is also secured with a pin. A third transcortical pin is placed near the distal extent of the osteotomy. Heavy gauge full cerclage wires are placed around the bone immediately proximal to each transcortical pin. Closure is routine.

77 Primary tenorrhaphy is the preferred method of tendon repair; however, this wound is highly contaminated which likely preclude performing a primary tenorrhaphy. If primary anastomosis is attempted, the contaminated wound should be adequately lavaged and debrided. Specimens should be obtained for culture and antimicrobial sensitivity, and broad-spectrum systemic antibiotic therapy should be initiated until results of the culture and sensitivity are available. In severely contaminated wounds repair may have to be delayed, and secondary tendon repair may be indicated. The wound should still be lavaged, debrided specimens obtained for culture and broad-spectrum antibiotic therapy initiated until results of the culture and sensitivity allow definite antibiotic selection. Monofilament non-absorbable sutures should be placed in the ends of the tendon segments for later identification. The wound should be treated with wet-to-dry dressings; tenorrhaphy can be performed at the time of wound closure or at a later date.

78 A drawing of an uniplanar, bilateral external skeletal fixator frame (78a).
i. What is the optimal number of pins that can be placed in each bone segment to maximize strength parameters of a bilateral frame?
ii. List two ways to significantly modify the strength and stiffness of this uniplanar-bilateral fixator–bone construct without changing the total number or size of pins or connectors?
iii. When a bilateral frame is applied to a non-load-sharing situation, what will be the weakest component of the construct counteracting axial compressive loads?
iv. Describe the single most substantial addition the surgeon can make to enhance the strength of this uniplanar-bilateral frame to resist axial compression, bending (in both the mediolateral and craniocaudal planes) and torsional disruptive forces.

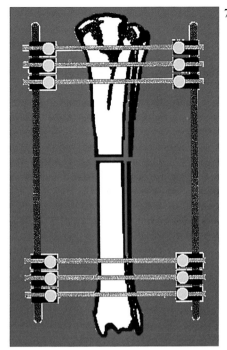

78a

79 Photographs illustrating a repair of a greater trochanteric fracture (79a, b).
i. What is the name of this fixation technique?
ii. Describe the biomechanical principle on which this technique is based?

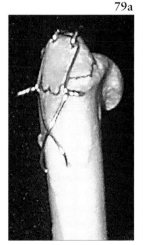

79a

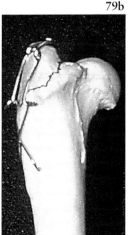

79b

78 i. In a study evaluating bilateral frame configurations, stiffness was augmented by increasing the number of pins up to four pins per bone segment. Placement of more than four pins per bone segment, however, did not significantly increase fixator–bone composite stiffness.

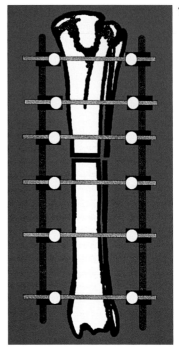

78b

ii. Spread out the fixation pins in each bone segment and decrease the connecting rod-to-bone distance. With this diaphyseal fracture, the fixation pins should be spread out evenly over each bone segment (78b). One pin in each segment should be placed close to the fracture site. The fracture site is the most devitalized region of the bone and the bone adjacent to the fracture site may contain microfissures. Pins should be placed at least 1 cm proximal and distal to the fracture site. These considerations become a trade-off of increasing mechanical stiffness versus the chance of stripping the pins and increasing the risk for infection.

iii. The fixation pins are the weakest component in a bilateral frame as opposed to a unilateral frame in which the connecting rod is the weakest component. Therefore, when axial compression is a concern with bilateral frames, the number (four per fracture segment being optimal) and size of the fixation pins should be maximized. In contrast, adding a second connecting rod or an intramedullary pin will improve the mechanical properties of a unilateral frame.

iv. A cranial uniplanar-unilateral type I frame can be added to make a biplanar-bilateral type III configuration. Type III configurations approach the strength of bone plates but offer the biologic advantage of not placing implants within the fracture site.

79 i. Tension band fixation.

ii. Sucessful fixation of this fracture requires a technique which opposes the distractive forces of the gluteal muscles and provides compression at the osteotomy. The figure-of-eight wire opposes the tensile forces produced by the gluteal muscles, resulting in a medially directed compressive force across the osteotomy. This resultant compressive force vector occurs because the proximally (tension produced by the gluteal muscles) and distally (resistance provided by the figure-of-eight wire) directed force vectors are not diametrically (180°) opposed. The Kirschner wires provide an anchor for the tension band wire and oppose shear forces while facilitating compression of the osteotomy. Ideally, the Kirschner wires should be oriented perpendicular to the osteotomy and placed parallel to each other.

80a

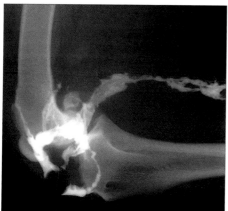

80b

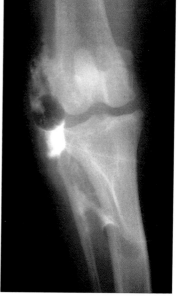

80 Lateral (80a) and craniocaudal (80b) views of a positive contrast fistulogram of the stifle region of an eight-year-old, spayed female Yorkshire Terrier that had an extra-capsular suture technique performed six months previously to stabilize its CCL defi-cient stifle. The dog became acutely non-weight-bearing on the limb three weeks ago and has a draining tract on the lateral aspect of the involved stifle.

i. What materials have been described for use as extracapsular 'sutures'? List advantages and disadvantages of each material.

ii. What anatomic placement of the suture results in the least change in the instant center of motion of the stifle joint?

iii. What complication has occurred in this dog, and how can the incidence of this complication be decreased?

81 A lateral view radiograph of the maxilla and mandible of a five-month-old Scottish Terrier presented with a history of anorexia and pain on opening the mouth of four weeks' duration (81a).

i. Describe the radiographic abnormalities and provide a diagnosis.

ii. What is the prognosis for this dog?

81a

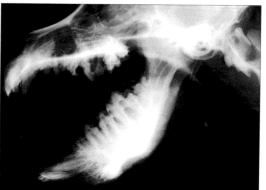

80 i.

Suture material	Advantages	Disadvantages
Monofilament nylon	High tensile strength Low reactivity Decreased bacterial colonization	Pre-sterilized, large-diameter material not available Difficult to handle
Multifilament non-absorbable suture	High tensile strength Available pre-sterilized in larger diameters	Higher reactivity Harbors bacteria, resulting in latent infections
Monofilament wire	High tensile strength Low reactivity	Requires wire passer Eventually breaks, resulting in transient lameness
Nylon band	High tensile strength Can apply without assistance	Biocompatibility untested Harbors bacteria, resulting in latent infections
Fascial strip	High biocompatibility No suture reaction	Marginal strength Recommended for dogs <15kg

ii. Placement of sutures from the lateral fabella to the tibial tuberosity does not change the instant center of motion of the stifle. Placement of sutures from the lateral fabella to the distal patellar tendon has been shown to change the normal motion of the stifle.
iii. Latent infection of the extracapsular suture (multifilament polyamide) resulting in a draining sinus. To minimize the incidence of this complication, non-reactive mono-filament suture material (i.e. nylon) can be used, or multifilament suture material may be soaked in chlorhexidine to inhibit bacterial colonization.

81 i. There is exuberent new bone formation which is limited to the horizontal
rami of both mandibles. Margins of the
new bone are slightly spiculated, indicating that the bone formation is still quite
active. These radiographic abnormalities
are characteristic of craniomandibular
osteopathy. This disease, of unknown
etiology, affects the flat bones of the skull,
especially the mandibles, tympanic bullae
and occipital bone. Craniomandibular
osteopathy is most often reported in Scot-

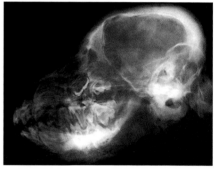

81b

tish and West Highland White Terriers, but isolated cases have also been reported in
Cairn and Boston Terriers, Labrador Retrievers, Great Danes, English Bulldogs and
Doberman Pinchers.
ii. A self-limiting disease, clinical signs are first noted at three to six months of age and
typically regresses at or before skeletal maturity. Only the mandibular rami are involved
in this dog, so the prognosis is good. Bony proliferation can be extensive, involving the
tympanic bullae and occipital bone, and can interfere with the temporomandibular joint
function (81b). The prognosis in dogs with more extensive involvement is guarded-to-
poor because the bony proliferation around the temporomandibular joints may make
eating and drinking impossible.

82 With regard to the Scottish Terrier in **81**, how should this dog's condition be treated?

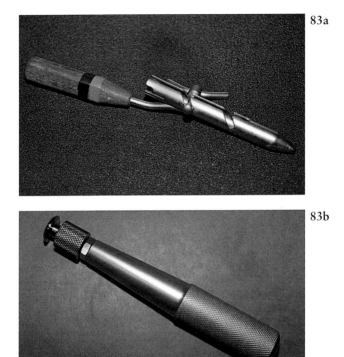

83a

83b

83 Photographs of two surgical instruments used to tighten cerclage wire (**83a, b**).
i. Describe the configuration of cerclage wire each of these instruments is designed to produce.
ii. What are the advantages and disadvantages of the two types of cerclage wires produced with these instruments?

82 Treatment is aimed at relieving pain and supporting the dog until the disease regresses. In mildly affected dogs, analgesics and hand feeding palatable foods may be the only treatment necessary. In severely affected dogs, feeding the dog via a pharyngostomy, esophagostomy or gastrostomy tube may be necessary because these dogs may be unable to eat or drink.

83 i. The instrument in 83a is used to tighten loop-type cerclage wires. The wire is placed around the bone and the free end of the wire is placed through the preformed eye of the wire, then through the oval hole in the end of the instrument and finally through the cannulation in the crank. The crank is placed in one of the paired slots in the instrument and turning the crank tightens the wire. When the wire is tight, the wire is secured by bending the wire through a 180° angle in the plane parallel to the loop (83c).

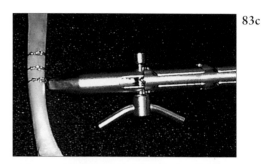

83c

The instrument in 83b is used to tighten twist-type cerclage wires. The instrument forms a braid as tightening and twisting of the knot are performed in one phase. The wire must be twisted while tension is applied to the instrument. This ensures that an even braid will be formed (83d).

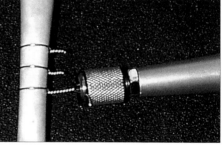

83d

ii. Although the *in vitro* static tension produced by loop-type cerclage wires is greater than twist-type cerclage wires, loop-type cerclage wires fail earlier than twist-type cerclage wires when subjected to loading. For all wire diameters tested, the twist-type cerclage wires have a greater ultimate strength and can sustain loads over a larger cerclage deformation than do the loop-type cerclage wires of the same wire diameter. This is attributed to the increased area of contact in the twist-type knot. The twist-knot pulls the wire through several planes, causing an increase in friction and resistance in the knot.

The protruding twist of the twist-type cerclage wires can irritate adjacent soft tissues; however, twist-type cerclage wires lose a significant amount of tension if the twist is bent over to lay against the cortex of the bone. Even cutting the twist-type wire causes a significant decrease in wire tension. Twist-type cerclage wires twisted until the wire breaks in the middle of the knot have greater tension than twist-type cerclage wires that are cut.

84 A photograph of a plastic femur with a simulated comminuted, mid-diaphyseal fracture, cut away to demonstrate stabilization with an intramedullary interlocking nail secured with four locking screws (84).
i. What are the indications for interlocking nailing in fracture stabilization?
ii. Why does interlocking nail fixation produce better fracture stability than intramedullary pin fixation?
iii. An alternative method of fracture stabilization in this type of fracture would be a plate applied in buttress fashion. What are the risks associated with buttress plating of comminuted diaphyseal fractures in comparison with stabilization with an interlocking nail?

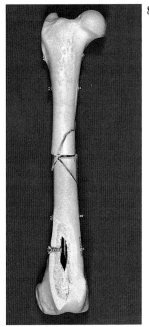

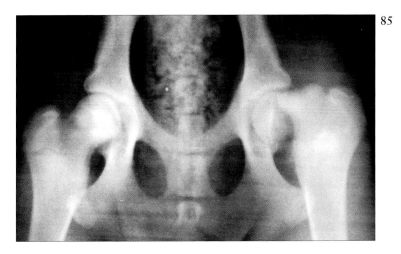

85 A ventrodorsal view radiograph of the pelvis of a four-month-old dog (85).
i. Describe the injury using the Salter–Harris classification scheme for physeal fractures.
ii. Describe the surgical techniques available for treatment of this type of fracture in dogs.

84 i. Interlocking nail fixation is indicated for stabilization of diaphyseal fractures of the femur, humerus and tibia. Fractures can vary in complexity from simple to comminuted; however, there must be at least 2–4 cm of intact diaphyseal–metaphyseal bone proximally and distally to allow for intramedullary insertion of the nail and placement of one or two locking screws.

ii. Intramedullary pin fixation provides excellent stability of fractures under bending loads, but not under rotational or axial loads. Only in cases of transverse or short oblique fractures, in which there is good interfragmentary bone contact, are fractures stable under axial loads. In these types of fractures the only resistance to rotational loads comes from interdigitation of the fractured bone segments, the surrounding cuff of periosteum and muscle, and friction between the pin and endosteal surface of the cortex. Interlocking nail fixation provides excellent stability under bending loads, similar to intramedullary pin fixation. Stability under both axial and rotational loads is also provided by the interlocking screws in the proximal and distal segments.

iii. A plate applied laterally in buttress fashion would be subjected to cyclic bending loads because the fracture segments of the medial *trans*-cortex are not in contact. This subjects the plate to cyclic bending forces and may lead to metal fatigue and failure of the plate before the fracture has healed. Because interlocking nails are positioned within the medullary cavity, which is in the neutral axis of loading, resistance to bending loads is greater than for a similar sized laterally applied plate. In addition, the area moment of inertia, and thus stiffness, of an 8 mm diameter nail is four times greater than a 3.5 mm broad DCP.

85 i. Salter–Harris type I fracture of the proximal femoral physis, often referred to as a femoral capital physeal fracture or a 'slipped capital physis.'

ii. Several surgical methods are described for repair of femoral capital physeal fractures. Several smooth Kirschner wires may be placed from just distal to the greater trochanter, through the femoral neck and into the capitus. These Kirschner wires are typically placed in a divergent fashion. Another technique is to place a bone screw from just distal to the greater trochanter through the femoral neck to engage the capitus. The screw is placed in lag fashion. A Kirschner wire is often used in conjunction with the screw to provide adjunctive rotational stability. Alternatively, two small bone screws can be placed through the articular surface of the capitus and into the femoral neck. The screw heads are countersunk below the cartilage surface. Biomechanical comparison of surgical methods found that fracture stabilization using a screw placed from the lateral surface of the femur or screws placed through the articular surface was significantly stronger than repair using Kirschner wires. Excision of the femoral head and neck may also be performed as a salvage procedure for femoral capital physeal fractures.

86 An intraoperative photograph of an autogenous cancellous bone graft harvested and placed at a fracture site (86).
i. What are the properties of a cancellous bone graft which promote bone union?
ii. List four indications for using an autogenous cancellous bone graft.
iii. List three cancellous bone donor sites which can be easily accessed in dogs.
iv. What complications are associated with the procurement of autogenous cancellous bone grafts in dogs?

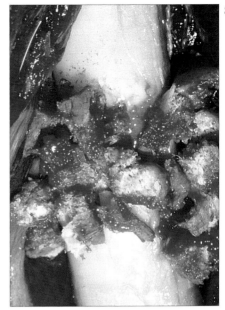

87 Lipid storage myopathies are best described in humans associated with either primary or secondary disorders of carnitine metabolism. Similar disorders have now been diagnosed in dogs. A composite of photomicrographs of a muscle biopsy from a dog with a lipid storage myopathy is shown (87).
i. What is the function of L-carnitine in muscle?
ii. What are typical presenting

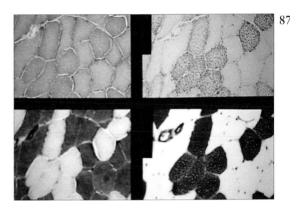

clinical signs in a dog affected with a lipid storage myopathy?
iii. What are the typical abnormalities observed in muscle biopsy specimens obtained from a dog with lipid storage myopathy?
iv. What specialized tests are necessary for a full analysis of these disorders?
v. What is the current treatment protocol for lipid storage myopathies?

86 i. Cancellous bone grafts have osteogenic, osteoinductive and osteoconductive properties. The osteogenic properties of cancellous bone grafts are attributed to surface cells of graft which survive the transplantation process and produce bone directly. Osteoinduction is the recruitment and differentiation of host mesenchymal cells by bone morphogenic proteins, osteogenin, osteoblast inductive factor, transforming growth factor-β and other bioactive growth factors. Osteoconduction describes the graft trabeculae serving as a scaffold or trellis for the migration of blood vesels and osteoblasts into the graft.
ii. (1) Promote bone union in the primary treatment of fractures, especially fractures with cortical bone loss. (2) Treatment of bone cysts. (3) Management of delayed, non-union, contaminated and infected fractures. (4) Accelerate union of arthrodeses.
iii. The proximal humerus, the proximal tibia and the wing of the ilium. These donor sites yield substantial amounts of cancellous bone and are easily approached. The specific donor site is chosen based on accessibility during surgery, quantity of graft required and the surgeon's personnal preference. Pre-operative planning is essential to insure the appropriate donor site(s) is prepared for surgery.
iv. Complications associated with harvesting autogenous cancellous bone graft are uncommon in dogs. Fracture of donor bone through the cortical defect has been reported. The potential for seeding the donor site with tumor cells or bacteria exists if the graft is not obtained as the initial procedure or with separate instruments.

87 i. L-carnitine is necessary for the transport of long-chain fatty acids across mitochondrial membranes; it is important in the enzymatically controlled degradation of fatty acids; and it has an important scavenging function in removal of toxic acyl compounds which at high concentrations interfere with energy production.
ii. Poorly localizable muscle pain, weakness and, if chronic, muscle atrophy. Orthopedic and neurologic evaluations, including myelography, do not result in a definitive diagnosis.
iii. Excessive lipid droplets within type I muscle fibers is usually the only abnormal finding (87, top left: modified trichrome stain showing vacuoles in some myofibers; top right: oil-red-O stain that identifies triglyceride droplets; bottom left: ATPase reaction pH 9.8 again identifying triglyceride droplets; bottom right: ATPase reaction pH 4.3 showing the localization of the lipid droplets to predominantly type I fibers).
iv. Specialized testing procedures include evaluation of plasma lactate/pyruvate ratios, evaluation of urine organic acids by gas chromatography/mass spectrometry, and quantitation of carnitine concentration in plasma, urine and muscle. Lactic and pyruvic acidemia are present in the majority of these cases supporting an underlying disorder of oxidative metabolism. Low muscle carnitine and increased excretion of urinary carnitine esters have also been found. These testing procedures are only available at laboratories specializing in the study of metabolic diseases.
v. If carnitine levels are low in muscle or there is increased urinary excretion of carnitine esters, supplementation with L-carnitine (50 mg/kg po bid) is recommended. Co-factor therapy including coenzyme Q10 (100 mg po daily) and riboflavin (100 mg po daily) has been recommended in humans and is currently being used in dogs.

88 A lateral view radiograph of the left femur of an 11-year-old, neutered male domestic shorthair cat with a two-day history of a left hindlimb lameness (88).
i. Describe the radiographic abnormalities.
ii. What is the recommended treatment?
iii. What is the prognosis?

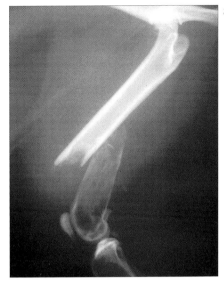

89 A lateral view radiograph of the left distal antebrachium of a five-month-old, male Irish Wolfhound with a history of a left forelimb lameness and mild valgus deformity of the left carpus (89).
i. What is the radiographic diagnosis?
ii. What is the pathogenesis of this condition?
iii. Which breeds of dogs are most commonly affected?

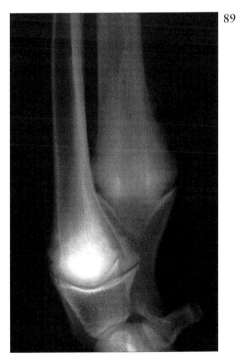

88 i. An oblique pathologic fracture of the distal femoral diaphysis; extensive intra-medullary and cortical lysis involving the distal fracture segment and the distal aspect of the proximal fracture segment; caudolateral displacement of the distal fragment with overriding. The primary lesion is most likely an appendicular osteosarcoma. Osteosarcomas occur relatively infrequently in cats. When diagnosed these tumors develop most commonly in the hindlimb of older, domestic shorthair cats. Radiographically these tumors typically involve the metaphyseal region of the long bones, and have a characteristic lytic (often described as a 'moth-eaten') appearance. Unlike osteosarcomas in dogs there is usually minimal periosteal reaction associated with osteosarcomas in cats.

ii. Amputation of the affected limb. The pre-surgical evaluation should include a complete blood count, chemistry profile, urinalysis and thoracic radiographs. Biopsies and aspirates of the affected site should be performed to confirm the diagnosis prior to definitive surgery. The cat should also be examined closely for regional lymph node involvement. An aspirate or biopsy of any affected lymph nodes should also be obtained to stage the disease process.

iii. The prognosis for cats with appendicular osteosarcoma is much better than that for dogs. Ninety per cent of dogs with appendicular osteosarcoma will die or be euthanized because of metastatic disease within four months following limb amputation. Adjunctive chemotherapy can increase the median survival time following limb amputation to approximately one year. The metastatic rate in cats with osteosarcoma following amputation in one study was less than 7% with a median survival time of greater than four years. The prognosis for cats with axial osteosarcoma does, however, differ significantly from cats with appendicular osteosarcoma. The median survival time for cats with axial osteosarcoma is reported to be five and a half months.

89 i. The dog has a retained cartilage core (RCC) associated with the distal ulnar physis and possibly retarded ulnar growth.

ii. RCCs (retained cartilage cores, retained endochondral cartilage cores) are caused by retarded endochondral ossification. RCCs are often bilateral, often clinically silent and may resolve uneventfully. The characteristic lesion is a cone-shaped mass of unmineralized hypertrophic cartilage with its base located at the center of the distal ulnar growth plate and its apex projecting into the metaphysis. The periphery of the physis is normal. The cause of the abnormality is unknown. One theory is that an interruption of oxygenation to a portion of the physis, perhaps due to microtrauma, results in an inability of the local environment to transform the cartilage into bone. While the distal ulnar physis is most commonly affected, RCCs have also been reported in the distal femur and distal tibia.

iii. Great Danes and Irish Wolfhounds. RCCs have also been reported in the Afghan, Collie and McKenzie Wolf. RCC is also reported in other species, including chickens, pigs and, possibly, horses.

90 With regard to the Irish Wolfhound in 89, what role does diet play in the etiology of this condition?

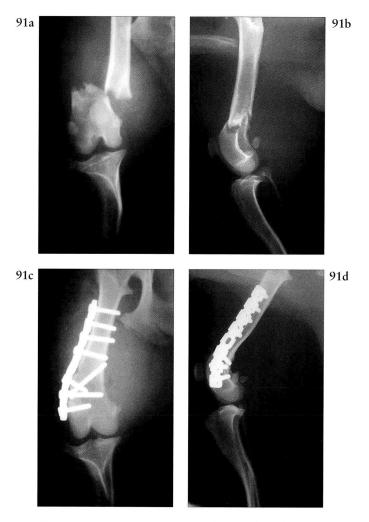

91a 91b 91c 91d

91 Pre-operative and post-operative craniocaudal and lateral view radiographs of the femur of a two-year-old Dachshund (91a–d).
i. Describe the fracture.
ii. What type of plate has been used to repair this fracture?
iii. Discuss the advantages and disadvantages of using this plate for this fracture.

90 RCC has been observed in Great Dane puppies fed several different types of diets; however, calcium levels specifically appear to affect the incidence of bone deformity associated with RCC. In a nutritional trial involving Great Dane puppies, 11/15 dogs studied developed RCC. None of these dogs developed angular limb deformities while on a calcium-controlled diet (1.1% dry matter basis). A high calcium diet (3.3% dry matter basis) resulted in RCCs being seen in 4/6 dogs, with two dogs developing subsequent severe angular limb deformity. A lower incidence (1/5) of RCC was found when Great Dane puppies were fed a very low calcium diet (0.57% dry matter basis); however, these dogs had a high incidence of distal radial compression fractures (4/5), presumably attributable to nutritional secondary hyperparathyroidism. Protein, energy content and level of exercise do not seem to play a role in the development of RCC.

91 i. A short oblique supracondylar femur fracture which is displaced cranio-laterally. Fractures involving the supracondylar region of the femur occur infrequently in skeletally mature dogs. Dogs with chondrodystrophoid conformation are predisposed to this type of fracture because the popliteal surface of the distal femur has a pronounced concavity.

ii. A reconstruction plate. Reconstruction plates were designed for mandibular reconstruction in humans. These plates are made of 316L stainless steel which is left in the annealed, or soft, condition which, combined with the notched design of the plate, facilitates three-dimensional contouring of the plate.

iii. Reconstruction plate fixation results in immediate rigid stabilization of the fracture. This allows early weight-bearing and offers a rapid and complete return of limb function. The notches between the holes of the reconstruction plate allow the plate to be bent in three dimensions, making it easier to contour the plate to the exaggerated caudal bow of this dogs' distal femur; the normal caudal bow of the distal femur is accentuated in dogs with chondrodystrophoid body conformation. This allows the surgeon to maximize the number of implant screws placed in the distal segment without interfering with stifle function as demonstrated on the cadaver femurs illustrated (91e). Reconstruction plates come in long lengths. A bolt cutter can be used to cut the plate at one of the notches to obtain a plate of the desired length. Reconstruction plates were not designed to withstand the forces of weight-bearing. The plate in this dog is functioning as a neutralization plate. A separate lag screw was placed outside the plate. Reconstruction plates are much less rigid than comparable sized DCPs and have a higher chance of bending failure, especially if the reconstruction plate is used to buttress large fracture gaps.

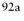
92a

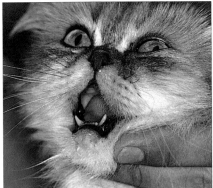

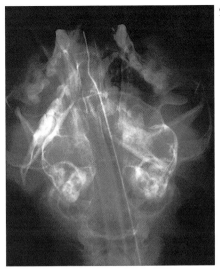
92b

92 A photograph of a two-year-old female Persian cat that is unable to close its mouth (92a). The cat has a two-month history of this problem occurring intermittently. The cat exhibits mild discomfort when the jaw is locked. A ventrodorsal view radiograph of the skull was made while the cat was unable to close its mouth (92b).
i. What is the most likely etiology of this problem?
ii. What is the surgical treatment of choice for this condition?

93 A photograph of a racing Greyhound with a muscular injury on the medial aspect of the left thigh just proximal to the stifle (93).
i. What muscle has been injured?
ii. What non-surgical treatments can be utilized in the first 48 hours following an injury such as this to reduce inflammation and hematoma formation?

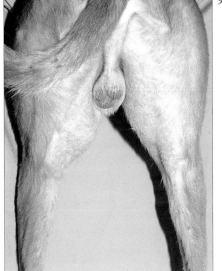
93

92 i. This cat has a condition which has been described as intermittent open mouth locking. The most common cause of this unusual condition is impingement of the coronoid process of the mandible on the ventral or lateral aspect of the zygomatic arch. Intermittent open mouth locking has also been reported in dogs with temporomandibular joint dysplasia without contact of the coronoid pro-

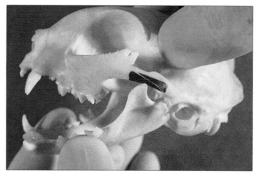

92c

cess with the zygomatic arch. Intermittent open mouth locking due to coronoid/zygomatic impingement has been reported in Persian cats and several breeds of dogs. This condition is usually associated with some degree of temporomandibular joint dysplasia with subsequent joint laxity and subluxation. Temporomandibular joint dysplasia might involve the bony structures or the soft tissue supportive elements of the joint, which includes the joint capsule, mandibular ligament and meniscus. Excess mandibular symphyseal laxity may also contribute to the lateral movement of the locking hemimandible. With sufficient laxity and lateral movement of the vertical ramus of the mandible, the coronoid process becomes hooked under the zygomatic arch. The radiograph shows obvious tilting of the mandible with impingement of the left coronoid process on the left zygomatic arch.

ii. Partial zygomatic arch resection has been described to treat this condition. Locking can be temporarily induced at surgery to identify the site of impingement. The portion of the zygomatic arch which impinges on the coronoid process, as defined in red on the skull shown (92c), is excised. Complete ostectomy of the involved zygomatic arch segment and/or resection of the coronoid process can be performed in animals with severe impingement.

93 i. The left gracilis muscle has been avulsed as evidenced by the swelling in the caudomedial region of the thigh. Avulsion of the gracilis muscle is one of the most common and serious muscular injuries affecting racing Greyhounds. If not repaired early, this injury usually ends a dog's racing career. The avulsion usually involves the caudal portion of the gracilis muscle and can occur at either the muscle's origin or the distal myotendinous junction.

ii. A cold compress, ice packs or cold spray should be applied to any muscle injury as soon as possible. Hypothermia causes vasoconstriction which reduces hematoma formation, swelling, edema and pain. Cold therapy should be applied for 15–20 minutes several times a day for the first 48–72 hours. A compressive bandage should be applied whenever possible. Restriction of movement and compression of the affected area helps to minimize inflammation and hematoma formation. Anti-inflammatory drugs can also be used to mitigate the inflammatory response.

94 With regard to the Greyhound in 93, how should surgical repair of this lesion be performed?

95 A photograph of a five-year-old, spayed female mixed-breed dog that was struck by a car and has a non-weight-bearing lameness of the left forelimb (95a). The elbow is flexed and the antebrachium is slightly abducted. Physical examination reveals pain, crepitus and decreased range of motion during manipulation of the left elbow joint. Radiographs of the elbow were obtained and a crainocaudal view radiograph of the left elbow is shown (95b).
i. What is the diagnosis?
ii. How should this condition be managed?
iii. What periarticular structures should be evaluated for structural damage?

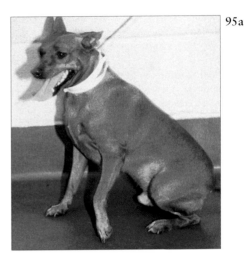

95a

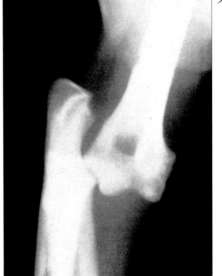

95b

94 Surgical repair of gracilis muscle injuries involves hematoma removal, muscle debridement and placement of appositional sutures. Apposition of the bulk of the muscle parenchyma can be achieved with pulley or large horizontal mattress sutures. Numerous small horizontal mattress or cruciate sutures can be used to appose the muscle sheath. Although some surgeons advocate the use of non-absorbable suture materials, excellent results have been achieved using polydioxanone and polyglycolic acid suture materials.

95 i. Traumatic lateral luxation of the left elbow. Concurrent fractures are not evident. The majority of elbow luxations are characterized by lateral or caudolateral displacement of the radius and ulna in relation to the humerus, because the large, sloping medial portion of the humeral condyle deters medial luxation.

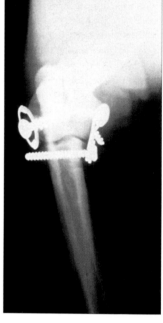

95c

ii. Most traumatic elbow luxations can be treated effectively by closed reduction if attempted within a few days of the injury. Orthogonal radiographs should be obtained to confirm the diagnosis and evaluate the joint for presence of fractures. The dog should be anesthetized to produce adequate muscle relaxation. The antebrachium is grasped and the elbow is held in 90–100° of flexion and the forelimb is internally rotated to reduce the luxation. Pressure is applied in a medial direction to the anconeal process until the anconeal process is positioned in the olecranon fossa. The elbow is then extended slightly while applying medial pressure to the proximal radius until the radial head is reduced. If closed reduction cannot be achieved, the dog should be prepared for surgery and an open reduction performed. Although some degenerative changes are expected to develop within the joint, the prognosis is favorable for luxations treated by closed reduction.

iii. The integrity of the collateral ligaments should be evaluated after reduction. This can be complicated by marked periarticular swelling in some dogs. The elbow should be flexed to 90° and the antebrachium pronated and supinated. The antebrachium can only be supinated to 45° and pronated 70° if the collateral ligaments of the elbow are intact. If the medial collateral ligament is disrupted, the antebrachium can be supinated to 140°. If the lateral collateral ligament is disrupted, the antebrachium can be pronated to 140°. Severe disruption of either ligament is indication for surgical repair. Repair of the collateral ligaments can be achieved by reattachment of an avulsed ligament using a screw and spiked washer or by replacement of the ligament by two screws and a prosthetic suture or wire (95c).

96a

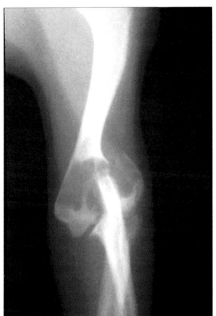

96b

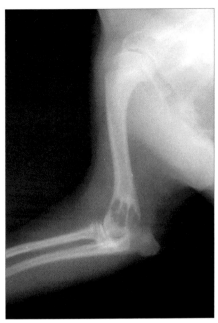

96 Radiographs of a six-month-old, intact female Yorkshire Terrier which developed a non-weight-bearing lameness two days prior to presentation (96a, b).
i. Describe the radiographic abnormalities.
ii. List the differential diagnoses for this lesion.
iii. What additional tests should be performed?
iv. What treatment options exist for this pathologic process?

97 A photograph of the hind quarters of a dog that has had a coaptation splint applied to its right hindlimb (97).
i. Name the coaptation splint.
ii. What is the primary indication for applying this type of coaptation splint?

97

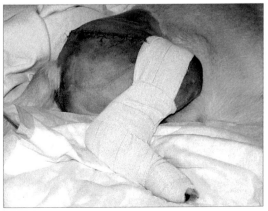

96 i. There is marked osteolysis of the distal humeral metaphysis with endosteal cortical lysis and absence of periosteal expansion. There is also a Salter–Harris type IV fracture involving the lateral portion of the humeral condyle with proximolateral displacement.

ii. The differential diagnoses include unicameral bone cyst, aneurysmal bone cyst, osteosarcoma, chondrosarcoma, osteomyelitis, fibrosarcoma, hemangioma, hemangiosarcoma, fibrous dysplasia (monostotic) and non-union fracture.

iii. Thoracic radiographs should be made and a biopsy of the osteolytic lesion obtained for histopathology as well as culture and sensitivity. In this dog the thoracic radiographs were normal and culture did not yield growth. Microscopic evaluation showed a thin layer of reactive periosteal bone and, within the lytic areas, extensive zones of hemorrhage with dilated, coalescent spaces filled with blood and hemosiderin-laden macrophages. Associated with this reaction was a variable cellular proliferation of reactive stellate multinucleated giant cells arranged in a stroma which varied from poorly cellular and edematous to densely cellular and fibrous. The multinucleated cells were most commonly identified in conjunction with delicate osteoid trabeculae of woven bone. There was no evidence of a concurrent neoplastic or infectious disease process. The radiographic and histologic findings in this dog were consistent with an aneurysmal bone cyst.

Three different types of bone cysts have been reported in dogs: subchondral, unicameral and aneurysmal. Subchondral cysts are believed to be a manifestation of osteochondrosis and are formed as a result of invagination of synovial membrane. Unicameral or simple bone cysts occur in young, large-breed dogs and are located in the metaphyseal area of long bones. Radiographically, the lesions are lytic and expansile. The cysts may be divided by a fibro-osseous septum and usually contain a straw-colored fluid or fibrous tissue. Aneurysmal bone cysts are expansive osteolytic lesions that develop secondary to hemodynamic alterations of the bone marrow. Benign and malignant neoplasia, fibrous dysplasia, unicameral bone cyst and trauma have been proposed as being inciting factors for aneurysmal bone cyst formation.

iv. Treatment options include curettage with or without cancellous bone grafting, cryotherapy, complete excision, irradiation or amputation. The latter was performed in this dog.

97 i. A 90–90 flexion splint.

ii. The 90–90 flexion splint is principally used to prevent fracture disease following open reduction and internal fixation of distal femoral fractures. Fracture disease, specifically 'quadriceps tie-down,' can be an unfortunate sequela to distal femoral fractures, particularly in skeletally immature dogs and cats. Fracture disease is most likely to develop if the limb is carried or coapted in extension following surgery. The 90–90 flexion splint is applied for five to ten days following surgery. The stifle and hock joints are positioned at approximately 90° of flexion by circumferentially wrapping elastic tape around the thigh and metatarsus, maintaining the quadriceps muscles in an extended position.

98 An immediate post-operative craniocaudal view radiograph of a right femur fracture in a domestic shorthair cat that was repaired with the combination of an intramedullary pin and a bone plate (98).
i. What is the term used to describe this concept of fracture management?
ii. Briefly describe the theory behind this method of fracture stabilization.

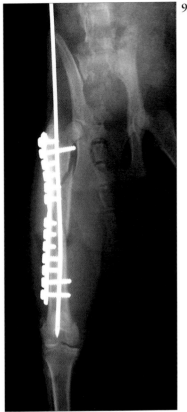

98

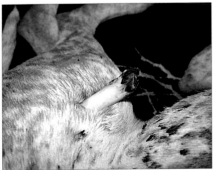

99a

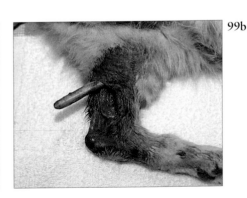

99b

99 Photographs of two different open fractures (99a, b). How are open fractures classified?

98 i. Biologic osteosynthesis.

ii. The concept of biologic osteosynthesis is based upon preservation of the soft tissue envelope and distribution of interfragmentary motion to a level which favors bone formation. Preservation of the surrounding soft tissue is maximized by the 'open but don't touch' (OBDT) technique. When managing comminuted fractures in this manner, spatial realignment of the limb is achieved by proper orientation of the proximal and distal bone segments without manipulating the comminuted bone fragments. The comminuted region of the fracture is buttressed with an appropriate implant, such as a bone plate, an interlocking intramedullary nail or an external fixator. The remaining large fracture gap distributes motion over a large area which lowers interfragmentary strain and promotes bone formation. In contrast, attempts to reduce highly comminuted bone fragments disrupts soft tissues and often leaves small fracture gaps where anatomic reduction is not possible. Movement in a small fracture gap concentrates strain and does not favor bone formation. Therefore, in a highly comminuted fracture such as this, the OBDT technique is favored since the soft tissue envelope is not disturbed and interfragmentary strain is low due to the large fracture gap. This fracture was managed with OBDT technique and combination plate/rod stabilization. A 2.0/2.7 mm veterinary cuttable plate was used. These plates are relatively weak. The empty screw hole over the comminuted region of the fracture serves as a stress concentrator and makes the plate susceptible to fatigue failure. Placement of the intramedullary pin extends the fatigue life of the plate. Biomechanical studies have determined that combining a bone plate with an intramedullary pin which occupies 50% of the diameter of the marrow cavity reduces the stress in the bone plate by one-half. Further, the fatigue life of the plate is extended 100 fold.

99 Open fractures have been classified based on the degree of soft tissue injury and contamination regardless of the underlying fracture. Wound classification provides prognostic information and guidance in the management of the injury. The following classification scheme proposed for use in companion animals by Tillson is a modification of the classification scheme proposed by Gustilo for use in humans:

- Type I: open fracture, small tissue laceration (<1 cm), minimal soft tissue trauma and contamination.
- Type II: open fracture, larger laceration (>1 cm), moderate soft tissue trauma, no flaps or avulsions, moderate contamination.
- Type IIIa: soft tissue available for wound coverage despite soft tissue laceration or flaps or high energy trauma, substantial contamination.
- Type IIIb: extensive soft tissue injury loss, periosteum stripped away from the bone and bone exposure, substantial contamination.
- Type IIIc: open fracture, arterial supply to the distal limb damaged, arterial repair required, substantial contamination.

100 With regard to the open fractures illustrated in 99, how would each of these be classified?

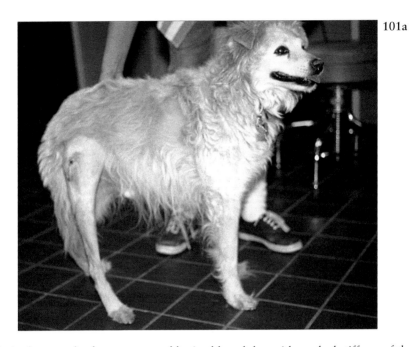

101a

101 A photograph of a seven-year-old mixed breed dog with marked stiffness of the hindlimbs and pain on palpation of the hindlimb musculature, which was tentatively ascribed to an endocrine-related myopathy (101a).
i. What common endocrinopathies can produce clinical signs of myalgia, stiffness, muscle weakness and muscle atrophy?
ii. What are the major effects that corticosteroids and thyroid hormone have on muscle?
iii. What pathologic changes are typically found within a muscle biopsy in a dog with Cushing's syndrome or hypothyroidism?
iv. Treatment of dogs with chronic exogenous corticosteroids may result in marked muscle weakness and muscle atrophy (so-called 'steroid myopathy'). What group of corticosteroids is reported to produce the most extensive muscle atrophy?

100 99a would be classified as a type II open fracture. This fracture was treated with surgical debridement and appropriate antibiotic therapy, and was stabilized with an intramedullary pin and 'tie-in' adjunctive external fixator. The fracture healed without complications. 99b would be classified as a type IIIb open fracture because there was extensive soft tissue damage and the periosteum was stripped away from much of the exposed tibia. Although this fracture was treated with surgical debridement and appropriate antibiotic therapy, and was anatomically reduced and rigidly stabilized with a bone plate, the segment of the tibia which had been stripped of its periosteum became infected and sequestered. The ensuing complications eventually led to amputation of the limb.

101 i. Hypothyroidism and Cushing's syndrome (both naturally occurring and iatrogenic) may have a myopathic presentation. Muscle stiffness, myalgia and weakness may be the only indication of an underlying endocrine disorder.
ii. Corticosteroid treatment impairs muscle protein and carbohydrate metabolism by decreasing protein synthesis, increasing protein degradation, decreasing amino acid uptake, altering glycolytic activity and producing insulin resistance. These effects are more pronounced in type 2 fibers than type 1 fibers. Muscle activity can alter the extent of GC induced muscle protein catabolism. Inactivity will exaggerate muscle atrophy produced by GCs and GC treatment will accelerate disuse atrophy. GC treatment will also intensify the catabolism of muscle protein associated with denervation. Thyroid hormone increases fatty acid oxidation, protein degradation and mitochondrial oxygen consumption. Hypothyroidism results in impaired energy metabolism and reduced protein turnover.

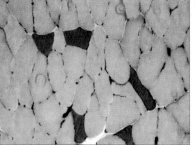

101b

101c

iii. The classical change found in muscle biopsies associated with excessive GC levels is selective atrophy of type 2 fibers. 101b is a histologic section (ATPase pH 9.8) of a muscle biopsy specimen obtained from a dog with 'steroid myopathy' induced by chronic GC administration for a skin disorder, showing atrophy of the darkly stained type 2 fibers. Hypothyroidism can produce an increase in the population of type 1 fibers. 101c is a histologic section (ATPase pH 9.8) of a muscle biopsy specimen obtained from a dog that was hypothyroid. Note the predominance of the lightly stained type 1 fibers. Although not present in these sections, myonecrosis can occur resulting in elevated serum creatine kinase.
iv. The fluorinated GCs (triamcinolone, betamethasone and dexamethasone) have been shown both in human and in experimental animal studies to have the highest myopathic potential.

102 Computerized force plate gait analysis can quantify limb function through the measurement of ground reaction forces. A force versus time curve for the fore- and hindlimbs of a dog at a trot is shown (**102a**).

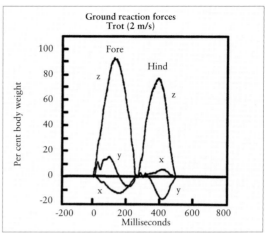

102a

i. What do the three orthogonal ground reaction forces (x, y, z) measure during force plate analysis. Which is the largest component of force in a dog at a trot?

ii. A significant linear correlation between ground reaction forces, impulses (force over time) and morphometric measurements (body weight, humeral length, femoral length and paw length) has been identified in dogs. Describe the relationship between morphometric characteristics and ground reaction force measurements in dogs.

iii. Numerous variables can affect the generation of ground reaction force and must be controlled when performing gait analysis to minimize variation. Name the causes of variance in gait analysis.

103 Photograph of cancellous bone that has been processed, double packaged in syringe cases, and stored at $-80°C$ ($-112°F$) (**103**). The cancellous bone is being thawed to be implanted as an allogenic cancellous bone graft in a dog with a highly comminuted tibial fracture.

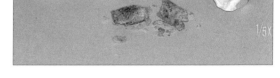

103

i. What are bone morphogenic proteins?

ii. Which bone morphogenic protein is purported to have the most potent osteoinductive effect?

iii. Does deep-freezing harvested cancellous bone have a detrimental effect on bone morphogenic proteins?

102, 103: Answers

102 i. Mediolateral force (Fx), braking/propulsion force (Fy) and vertical force (Fz). Vertical force is the largest component of force (102b).

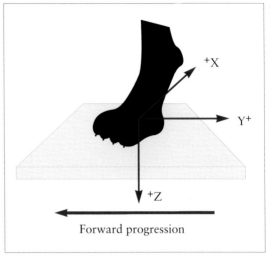

102b

ii. Impulse is the total force applied over a period of time and is directly correlated with physical size. Peak force is the maxium force applied during a stance phase and is inversely correlated with physical size. Thus, larger dogs apply less peak force to their limbs but apply force over an increased time (longer stance phase). The longer stance phase spreads the impulsive forces over more time, decreasing the peak loads applied to the musculoskeletal system. Larger dogs also require a greater braking force to stop a limb's forward motion and a greater propulsive impulse to initiate the next stride. Because of this relationship between morphometeric measurements and ground reaction forces, comparisons of force plate data are only valid if the dogs have similar morphometric characteristics.

iii. Changes in subject velocity; handler differences; trial variation for each subject; sensitivity of the force plate; inherent subject variation; morphometric differences between subjects; and limb acceleration and deceleration.

103 i. Bone morphogenic proteins are bone matrix components thought to induce mesenchymal cell differentiation along the osteoblast line. The bone morphogenic proteins are differentiative (osteoinductive), but have no mitogenic effect (osteogenic). Nine different bone morphogenic protein molecules have been identified to date. Bone morphogenic proteins are a part of a complex interaction of cytokines and growth hormones involved in bone healing. Bone grafts release bone morphogenic proteins which cause precursor cells to differentiate and become osteoblasts. This osteoinductive property makes bone grafts superior to most bone substitutes for resolving bone defects.

ii. Bone morphogenic protein-2 (rhBMP-2) is currently considered to be the most potent of the bone morphogenic proteins. Most clinical and experimental investigations have focused on rhBMP-2. Bone morphogenic protein-7 (rhBMP-7) is also being evaluated for clinical applications, despite it having inferior potency to rhBMP-2.

iii. Deep-freezing bone to −80°C (−112°F) is not thought to have an appreciable adverse effect of the osteoinductive potency of bone morphogenic proteins.

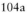

104a

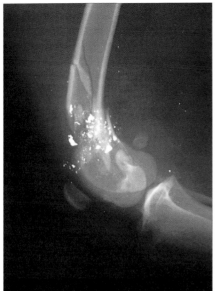

104b

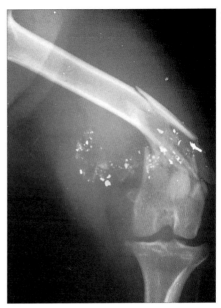

104 Lateral (**104a**) and craniocaudal (**104b**) view radiographs of the distal femur of a three-year-old, neutered male Labrador Retriever that was presented for treatment of a comminuted distal femoral fracture sustained as a result of a gunshot injury. There were no discernable neurovascular deficits.
i. Describe the fracture.
ii. What types of bone plates could be used to stabilize this fracture?

105 Photograph of a cat's distal humerus (**105**).
i. Give the name of the foramen in the center of the circle.
ii. What anatomic structures pass through this foramen?

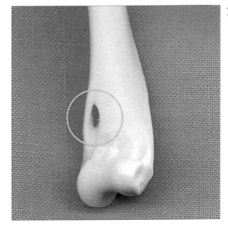

105

104c 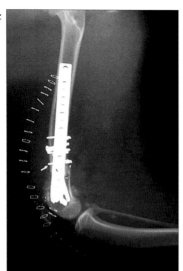 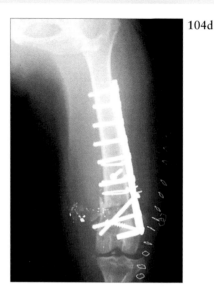 104d

104 i. The supracondylar region of the left femur is highly comminuted. There are several large lateral butterfly fragments and medial angulation of the distal fragment. There are numerous metal densities indicative of a gunshot wound. This fracture would be classified as a type III gunshot injury, characterized by severe comminution with cortical defects and extensive soft tissue trauma. Type I gunshot injuries are simple fractures with minimal soft tissue damage, whereas type II gunshot injuries are severely comminuted but without cortical defects and extensive soft tissue damage.

ii. A DCP could be used to stabilize this fracture. Because the fracture involves the supracondylar region of the femur, it would be difficult to place three screws in the distal fracture segment if a DCP were used. Reconstruction plates have been used to stabilize supracondylar femoral fractures. These plates allow three-dimensional contouring which can facilitate placement of an additional screw in the distal femoral segment; however, the design and greater ductility of reconstruction plates decreases these plates' bending stiffness. Reconstruction plates are inadequate to buttress large metaphyseal defects and would likely fail if used to stabilize this dog's fracture. This fracture was repaired using a customized hook plate constructed by modifying a 3.5 mm DCP (**104c, d**). The hook plate provides two additional points of fixation where use of a standard DCP would not allow three screws or six cortices of purchase. The customized hook plate allows greater flexibility in choosing the length of the plate. Manufactured hook plates are not available in adequate lengths to properly stabilize this dog's combined supracondylar and diaphyseal fracture.

105 i. The supracondylar foramen.
ii. The median nerve and brachial artery.

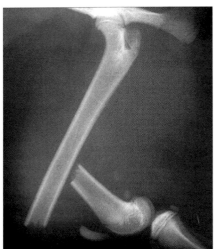

106a

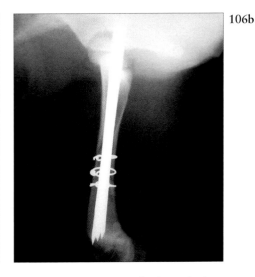

106b

106 Pre-operative (**106a**) and immediate post-operative (**106b**) lateral view radiographs of the femur of a seven-month-old mixed-breed dog which was stepped on by a horse.
i. What biomechanical forces created this fracture?
ii. Why were multiple intramedullary pins used instead of a single intramedullary pins?
iii. What purpose are the cerclage wires serving, and what other adjunctive fixation could be used to stabilize this fracture?

107 A lateral view radiograph of the stifle of a four-month-old, male Greyhound with a two-day history of a non-weight-bearing right hindlimb lameness (**107**). Physical examination revealed pain and crepitus with flexion and extension of the affected stifle joint. Swelling was also evident in the area of the insertion of the straight patellar ligament.
i. What lesion is present on this radiograph?
ii. What two related injuries have been reported to accompany the lesion seen on this radiograph?
iii. What are the treatment options for this condition?

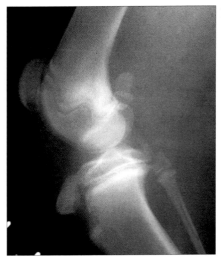

107

106 i. Transverse fractures, like the fracture in this dog, are created when the loading forces are concentrated at a point perpendicular to the long axis of the bone. Cortical bone displays a viscoelastic response to loading and will fail under relatively low loads when loaded slowly. Conversely, cortical bone exhibits greater stiffness when loaded rapidly and thus is capable of absorbing more energy before ultimate failure. Simple transverse fractures occur when loading forces are applied slowly to a bone as occurred in this dog.

ii. A single intramedullary pin offers little resistance to torsional forces. Stack pinning is a useful technique to improve torsional stability. Three or more smaller pins are selected which fill the medullary canal at the isthmus. In one *in vivo* study, multiple intramedullary pins provided approximately twice the rotational resistance of a single intramedullary pin. Complications can arise following single or multiple intramedullary pin stabilization if case selection is not carefully scrutinized prior to surgery. Adjunctive fixation should be considered with any intramedullary pinning procedure.

iii. Cerclage wires were used in this fracture because fissures were propagating in the proximal fracture segment. The cerclage wires do not provide any rotational stability. Hemicerclage wire techniques do not provide sufficient torsional stability and would be inappropriate for use in this dog because of the presence of the fissures. If the placement of multiple intramedullary pins did not provide sufficient rotational stability in this dog, consideration should have been given to using an adjunctive type I external fixator. An adjunctive two pin, single connecting rod type I external fixator has been shown to provide significantly greater torsional resistance than multiple intramedullary pins.

107 i. The apophysis of the tibial tuberosity is avulsed and displaced cranially and proximally, and the patella is located more proximal than normal. Tibial tuberosity avulsions vary in severity from minimally displaced 'partial' avulsions to severe 'complete' separation of the apophysis from the metaphysis of the tibia. Radiographs of the contralateral stifle may be necessary to diagnose minimally displaced avulsions.

ii. Fracture of the distal patella accompanies avulsion of the tibial tuberosity in approximately 15% of Greyhounds. Fracture/separation of the proximal tibial epiphysis may also occur with tibial tuberosity avulsion.

iii. Tibial tuberosity avulsions can be managed with or without surgical intervention. Conservative treatment is appropriate when there is minimal displacement of the apophysis or in dogs with chronic avulsions which have begun to heal and are palpably stable, particularly if pain and lameness are no longer present. Conservative therapy usually consists of three weeks of cage rest. A modified Robert Jones bandage may be applied for the first seven days. Open reduction and internal fixation are indicated in acute, moderately-to-severely displaced avulsions and in dogs with distal patellar fractures. Chronic avulsions which are severely displaced or remain painful can also be treated surgically. Implants used for internal fixation include small diameter Steinmann pins or Kirschner wires with or without a figure-of-eight tension band wire, Kirschner wires, lag screw, wire suture and Smillie and Stille nails. Fixation with two Kirschner wires is preferred. Early removal of implants (e.g. two to three weeks), particularly those which compress the growth plate, is recommended, especially in very young patients.

108 With regard to the Greyhound in 107, what complications may be seen with surgical treatment of this condition?

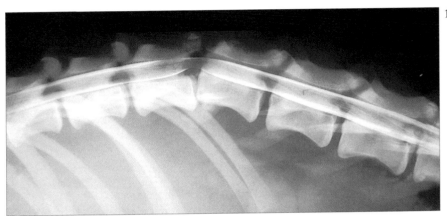

109a

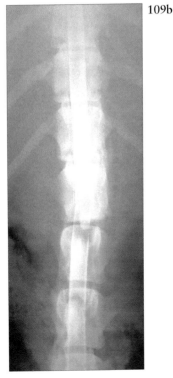

109b

109 Lateral (109a) and ventrodorsal (109b) view positive contrast myelographic studies of the thoracolumbar vertebral column of a three-year-old, female Pointer that was hit one month ago by a car. The dog was initially treated with confinement in a cage but is still non-ambulatory paraparetic with upper motor neuron signs in both hindlimbs. Deep pain perception is present in the tail and both hindlimbs and the dog is continent.
i. Describe the radiographic abnormalities.
ii. Discuss appropriate surgical decompression and stabilization of this injury.

108 Non-union of the tibial tuberosity secondary to implant failure. Techniques which compress the growth plate (e.g. lag screw or tension band fixation) may result in flattening and distal translocation of the tuberosity (108).

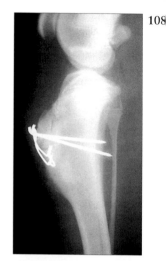

108

109 i. There is a fracture/luxation at L1-L2. The L1-L2 intervertebral disc space is narrowed and there is dorsolateral displacement of L2. There is periosteal bone formation at the cranioventral aspect of the vertebral body of L2. The contrast column is attenuated at the L1-L2 articulation.

ii. The two issues to be considered are decompression and stabilization techniques. Unless there is disc material or a displaced bone fragment in the spinal canal, decompression can generally be achieved by realigning the fracture/ luxation. Exploratory laminectomies or hemilaminectomies further destabilize the vertebral column and are generally avoided; however, a left hemilamenectomy was done in this dog to assist in the visual assessment of reduction. In order to properly immobilize vertebral column injuries, it is necessary to bridge the unstable site with fixation that engages solid bone both cranial and caudal to the injury. The segment of spine that is immobilized by the apparatus should be as short as possible. The apparatus should be inert and biocompatible to avoid complications and the need for implant removal. In this dog, unilateral vertebral body fixation pins and a PMMA column were used to stabilize the fracture/luxation (109c, d). Vertebral body plating techniques could have also been used in this region of the spine. Although bench research studies indicate that a biomechanical advantage can be gained through the simultaneous use of more than one form of fixation, such as combining vertebral body stabilization with articular facet or dorsal spinous process stabilization, versatility and clinical success has led many surgeons to use vertebral body fixation pins and PMMA to stabilize unstable vertebral segments.

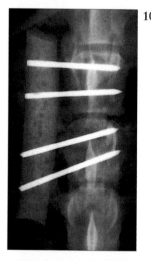

109

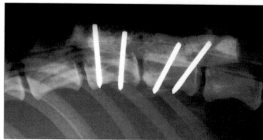

109

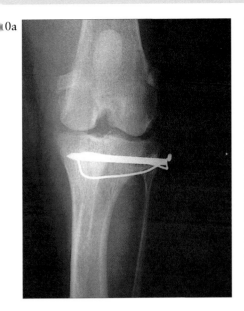

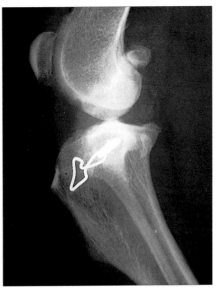

110 Craniocaudal (110a) and lateral (110b) view radiographs of the stifle of a two-year-old, intact male Rottweiler that had surgery three weeks previously because the dog had sustained a CCL injury. The dog had since developed a fluid-filled swelling distal and lateral to the stifle.
i. Based on the radiographs, what procedure was used to stabilize this dog's stifle?
ii. What anatomic structure is used to resolve the instability in the CCL deficient stifle with this technique?
iii. What are the major complications associated with this method of stabilizing the CCL deficient stifle?

111 An unstained cross-section of cortical bone in the femoral diaphysis under UV illumination (×200) (111).
i. Identify the structures with the concentric fluorescent rings.
ii. What is bone (mineral) apposition rate, and how is it measured?

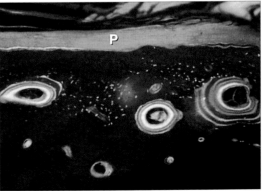

110 i. A fibular head transposition was performed. The fibular head is freed from the tibia, advanced cranially, and a Steinmann pin or Kirschner wire is placed in the caudal portion of the fibular head and seated in the tibia. The orthopedic wire twisted around the pin extends through two bone tunnels in the tibial crest, maintaining the fibular head in the advanced position.

ii. The fibular head transposition is an extracapsular technique which re-establishes stifle stability by cranial advancement of the bone–ligament unit consisting of the lateral collateral ligament of the stifle and the fibular head. This limits cranial drawer and internal rotation of the tibia on the femoral condyles.

iii. In one retrospective study the most common complication associated with this procedure was iatrogenic fracture of the fibular head. Fracture of the fibular head occurs when the fibular head has not been entirely freed from its syndesmotic attachment to the tibia or results from cranial placement of the Steinmann pin or Kirschner wire in the fibular head. If fracture occurs, continued instability will result. The Steinmann pin or Kirschner wire should, therefore, be placed in the caudal portion of the fibular head. Inadequate advancement of the fibular head results in persistent stifle instability. Stifle instability should be assessed at surgery and, if still present, the fibular head should be advanced further cranial until the stifle is stable. Although accidental transection of the lateral collateral ligament can occur while freeing the fibular head from its syndesmotic attachment, the frequency of this complication has not been reported. Directing the scalpel blade from proximal to distal is recommended to help prevent iatrogenic transection of the lateral collateral ligament. Implant loosening can occur and has been associated with seroma formation and discomfort in the limb. If the lameness persists, implant removal may resolve the resulting pain. Although a number of complications can occur with this technique, successful clinical outcomes associated with fibular head transposition are reported to be greater than 90%.

111 i. The fluorescent rings indicate the presence of forming osteons (Haversian systems) near the outer or periosteal (P) surface of cortical bone. Fluorochrome compounds such as tetracycline derivatives and calcein bind to calcium and are deposited in new bone matrix (osteoid) as it rapidly calcifies soon after its initial deposition by osteoblasts. Therefore, fluorochrome compounds label bone forming surfaces. When viewed under UV illumination, they fluoresce brightly and serve as an important research tool for measurements of osteoblast activity and bone formation rates. The presence of bone forming osteons is characteristic of cortical bone remodeling. In this process, old bone with microdamage is first removed by osteoclasts and subsequently replaced with new bone deposited by osteoblasts. Thus, the resorption cavities in cortical bone are eventually filled with new bone to form a completed osteon with a central Haversian canal surrounded by concentric lamellae. In a cross-section of cortical bone, both resorption cavities and forming osteons in various stages of filling the resorption cavities are usually observed.

ii. The distance between two fluorochrome labels can be measured and divided by the time interval between their administration to calculate a bone (mineral) apposition rate. The resulting value is indicative of the rate at which osteoblasts deposit new bone matrix.

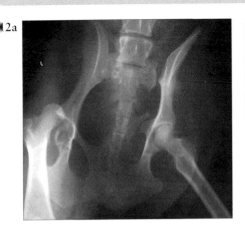

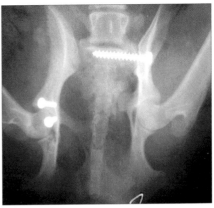

112 A ventrodorsal view radiograph of the pelvis of an eight-year-old Miniature Schnauzer which had been hit by a car (112a). The dog was unable to bear weight on either hindlimb due to coxofemoral luxation and contralateral sacroiliac fracture–luxation. This dog's sacroiliac fracture–luxation was reduced and stabilized in order to hasten the dog's recovery (112b).

i. In one study, 38% of sacroiliac fracture–luxations repaired by lag screw fixation experienced premature screw loosening. Dogs with the lag screws placed into the sacral body had the lowest rate of loosened fixations. Describe the anatomic landmarks on the sacral wing which can be used by the surgeon to locate the sacral body for screw placement.

ii. What has been determined to be the optimum depth of screw placement into the sacral body in order to minimize implant loosening?

iii. Combinations of pins and screws have been used to stabilize sacroiliac fracture–luxations. Rank the implant combinations used to repair sacroiliac fracture–luxation in order of increasing stability.

113 A photograph of an adjunctive 'tie-in' external skeletal fixator that was used to stabilize a comminuted diaphyseal fracture of the humerus (113).

i. What material is used most often to form the acrylic column?

ii. List six advantages of using acrylic connecting columns.

iii. List three disadvantages of using acrylic connecting columns.

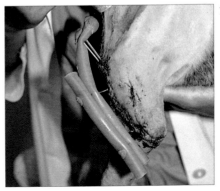

112 i. The sacral body can be located by identifying the notch that is present along the cranial edge of the sacral wing. A screw placed just caudal to this notch will be within the sacral body. If this notch is not palpable, the sacral body can be located by identifying the most craniodorsal and ventral aspects of the sacral wing. An imaginary line is drawn between these two points. The sacral body is located by estimating a point 60% of the distance from the craniodorsal aspect to the ventral most aspect of the sacral wing. The screw should be placed just caudal to this point to be in the sacral body. A final guide is to position the screw hole 2 mm cranial and 2 mm dorsal to the center of the crescent-shaped, semilunar, articular cartilage on the sacral wing.
ii. The cumulative screw depth should be at least 60% of the sacral body width. Therefore, if a single screw is used, the screw should transverse 60% of the sacral width. If two screws are used, the combined depth of both screws should total at least 60% of the sacral width.
iii. A single screw accurately placed into the sacral body gives equal fixation strength when compared to a screw and a Kirschner wire. Placement of two screws provides superior stability to a single screw or a single screw plus a Kirschner wire. In all instances, use of the largest diameter screw possible maximizes the stability of the repair and all screws must be placed in lag fashion.

113 i. PMMA. The columns are often applied following fixation pin placement and wound closure, usually after post-operative radiographs have confirmed proper reduction and fixation pin placement. Thus non-sterile, non-medical grade PMMA is often used because it is much less expensive than sterile, medical grade PMMA.
ii. (1) The diameter of the fixation pins is not restricted to those pins that can be accommodated by connecting clamps. Any diameter fixation pin can be used. This is very important when using a 'tie-in' configuration, as depicted in this case, because multiple small diameter intramedullary pins were used. (2) Fixation pin placement need not be linear to conform to a straight, rigid connecting rod. Fixation pins can be placed in multiple planes. (3) The acrylic column can be modeled to conform to the contours of the limb, decreasing the distance between the *cis*-cortex of the bone and the connecting column. Decreasing the distance between the connecting column and the *cis*-cortex substantially increases the stiffness of the bone–fixator construct. (4) Most acrylics (unless barium sulfate has been added) are radiolucent which facilitates post-operative radiographic assessment of fracture reduction and subsequently fracture healing. (5) Acrylic columns are lightweight which encourages an early return of limb function, particularly in smaller animals. (6) Acrylic connecting systems are also very economical.
iii. (1) Reduction can be difficult to maintain if acrylic connecting columns are used as primary stabilization. The lack of fixator rigidity prior to polymerization of the acrylic makes acrylic connecting columns better suited for adjunctive fixation. (2) Post-operative adjustments, as necessitated by excessive soft tissue swelling or fixation pin complications, are much more difficult to make than with standard metal connecting systems. (3) The fumes released during polymerization of the methylmethacrylate are noxious and toxic.

114 A positive contrast arthrogram of the scapulohumeral joint of a three-year-old German Shepherd Dog which was treated for OCD of the humeral head two years previously by an arthrotomy and removal of a fragmented cartilage flap (114a). The dog's lameness has persisted since surgery.
i. What is the reason for the dog's persistent lameness?
ii. Could this condition have been diagnosed prior to the initial surgery?
iii. What is the incidence of this sequela to OCD of the humeral head?

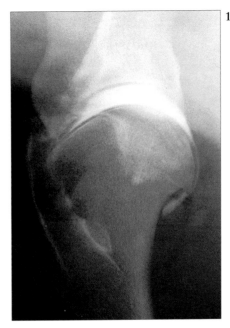
114a

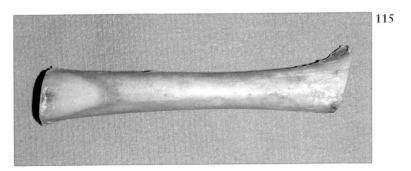
115

115 A photograph of a cortical bone alloimplant which has been harvested and prepared for banking (115).
i. List three methods of preparing and storing cortical bone for future use as a cortical alloimplant.
ii. How do properly implanted cortical bone allografts function when used to resolve large diaphyseal bone defects?

114 i. The cartilage lesion of the original OCD lesion has been replaced with fibrous repair tissue, but there is a filling defect in the contrast media present within the caudodistal bicipital tendon sheath (114b, arrow). The filling defect is caused by a cartilage fragment (or 'joint mouse'), which detached from the OCD lesion and migrated into the bicipital tendon sheath. Cartilage fragments that lodge in the bicipital tendon sheath cause mechanical irritation and tenosynovitis, leading to pain and lameness. Surgical removal of the 'joint mouse' lodged in the bicipital tendon sheath is indicated.

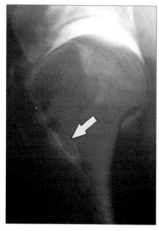

11

ii. Perform a pre-operative, positive-contrast arthrogram. Positive-contrast arthrography is accurate in detecting detached cartilage fragments or 'joint mice,' especially within the bicipital tendon sheath.

iii. Approximately 10%. Detection of cartilage fragments clearly requires arthrography unless the fragments become mineralized. In one study only 10% of detached cartilage flaps lodged in the bicipital tendon sheath were visible on plain radiographs; however, all were demonstrated by positive-contrast arthrography.

115 i. (1) Sterile harvested, frozen bone is the standard preparation for cortical bone banked for future use. Donors must be screened for infectious diseases. The donor is euthanized (or anesthetized until the bone is harvested and then euthanized) and multiple donor sites prepared for aseptic harvest. All soft tissues are removed to decrease the antigenicity of the implant. Bones are double wrapped before storage. Freezing the bone at –20°C (–4°F) appears sufficient to store bone and retain mechanical properties successfully. Recommended length of safe storage time varies from six months (recommended by the American Association of Tissue Banks) to two years. Bone stored at –70°C (–94°F) can be stored up to five years. (2) Freeze-drying is used extensively for storing bone in human medicine. Bones are harvested aseptically as previously described. After freeze-drying the bone can be stored at room temperature. The process requires lyophilization equipment and can be expensive. Tissue must be rehydrated prior to use and may have less than ideal mechanical properties. (3) Alternatively, unscreened donors are euthanized. The bone is harvested and the soft tissues removed without aseptic surgical precautions. The bone is double wrapped and sterilized with ethylene oxide. The bone is aerated to remove the residues of ethylene oxide and is stored at –20°C (–4°F). There are mixed reviews from the literature concerning the compatibility of ethylene oxide sterilized tissue with the host.

ii. Cortical bone grafts treated with these protocols act as weight-bearing struts, providing mechanical stability. Cortical bone grafts also serve as scaffolds for the ingrowth of new host bone, providing an osteoconductive property.

116 A lateral radiograph of the right
carpus of a two-year-old, male racing
Greyhound with a type I fracture of the
accessory carpal bone (116a).
i. Which soft tissue structures are associated with the small bone fragment
(arrow) fractured off the distal margin of
the articular surface?
ii. What are the sequelae if this type of
fracture is not treated surgically?
iii. Describe two methods of surgical
treatment for this fracture.

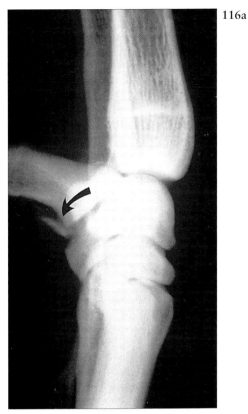

116a

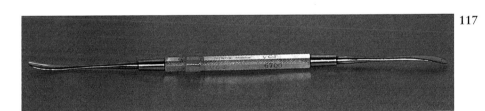

117

117 Name the surgical instrument illustrated (117).

116b

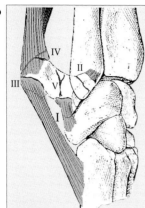

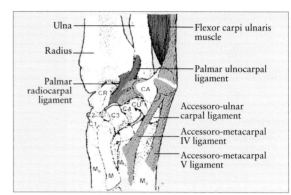

116

116 i. Fractures of the accessory carpal bone are a common injury in racing Greyhounds. Most occur in the right carpus due to the stress of racing on circular or oval tracks in a counterclockwise direction. These fractures have been classified into five types (116b). This dog has a type I fracture. The accessoro-ulnar carpal ligament and joint capsule insert in this region of the accessory carpal bone, and form part of the ligamentous support of this articulation between the accessory carpal and ulnar carpal bones (116c).

116d

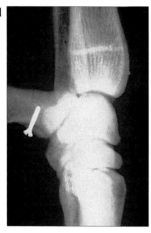

ii. This is an intra-articular fracture. Osseous union rarely occurs without surgical intervention because of instability and because synovial fluid enters the fracture line. Chronic fractures cause abrasion of the articular cartilage of the proximal aspect of the ulnar carpal bone and osteoarthritis.

iii. (1) Internal fixation of the fracture with a screw. Open reduction and internal fixation are performed via a caudolateral approach. The abductor digiti quinti muscle is reflected at its origin and the fracture fragment is found deep to the two accessoro-metacarpal IV and V ligaments that connect to metacarpal bones IV and V. Fracture reduction is maintained with small pointed reduction forceps. Internal fixation of the fracture is performed with a 1.5 or 2 mm cortical bone screw (116d). One study found that of 12 racing greyhounds with fractures repaired by screw fixation, ten dogs returned to racing and five dogs won one or more races. (2) Excision of the avulsed fragment is performed via the same approach. After fragment excision, no attempt is made to repair the damaged accessoro–ulnar carpal ligament and healing proceeds by fibroplasia. One study found that of 19 racing greyhounds treated by this method, 13 dogs returned to racing and nine won races.

117 A Freer periosteal elevator.

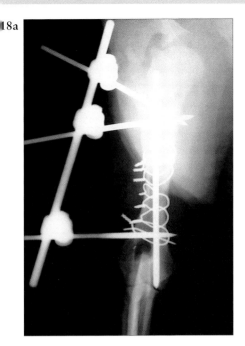
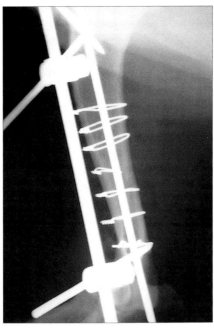

118 Immediate post-operative radiographs of a humeral fracture in a three-year-old, female mixed-breed dog that was repaired using multiple cerclage wires, an intramedullary Steinmann pin and an adjunctive external fixator (118a, b). What are the basic principles of proper cerclage wire application?

119 Two DCPs (bottom) and two limited contact DCPs (top) (119).
i. What material was used to make the DCPs pictured here? What are the constituents that make up this material?
ii. What material was used to make the limited contact DCPs pictured here? What are the constituents that make up this material?
iii. Compare the material property differences of the DCPs and the limited contact DCPs pictured here.

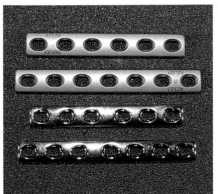

118 Cerclage wires should be used in conjunction with other implants, never as primary fixation for the stabilization of long bone fractures. Cerclage wires maintain fragment apposition but are only suitable for providing adjunctive fixation to counteract the bending, shear, torsional and axial loads associated with weight-bearing.

Full 360° anatomic reconstruction of the circumference of the bone at the level of wire application is mandatory.

The wire must be of sufficient (generally 18 or 20 gauge) diameter.

Multiple wires, rather than a single wire, should be placed. A single cerclage wire placed at a fracture site will act as a fulcrum, concentrating bending forces at the fracture site.

Cerclage wires should be used for oblique fractures to produce interfragmentary compression. The length of the fracture line should be at least twice as long as the diameter of the bone at the level of wire application. Application of cerclage wires to short oblique fractures produces shear rather than compressive forces.

Cerclage wires should be placed 10 mm apart and at least 5 mm from the transverse portion of the fracture. Wires should not be placed in the fracture line.

Cerclage wires should be placed perpendicular to the long axis of the bone. If the wire is placed obliquely to the long axis of the bone, the diameter of the wire loop will exceed that of the bone. The cerclage wire will eventually shift and become loose, impeding vascularization and fracture healing.

In regions where the bone is changing shape or diameter, measures must be taken to prevent the cerclage wire from slipping. Consideration should be given to using a hemicerclage wire, placing the wire in notches made in the cortices of the bone or placing a Kirschner wire subjacent to the cerclage wire to prevent slippage.

Cerclage wires must be tight after application. Soft tissues should not be interposed between the wire and bone; however, excessive dissection of soft tissues during application of the wire should be avoided. Using a wire passer greatly facilitates proper wire placement.

119 i. 316L stainless steel. The constituents of stainless steel includes approximately 18% chromium, 10–14% nickel, 2–4% molybdenum, and several other inert elements (i.e. carbon, manganese, sulfur and phosphorus). The remainder of the material is made up of iron (approximately 55–60%). The 'L' designates low carbon content.
ii. Pure titanium. Pure titanium is less brittle, unlike titanium alloy which is made up of 90% titanium, 6% aluminum and 4% vanadium, and has mechanical properties more similar to cold-worked stainless steel.
iii. Titanium in a pure form is extremely resistant to corrosion. Titanium is able to form an oxide layer spontaneously which limits corrosion in a saline solution and may make this implant material more resistant to corrosion than stainless steel. Furthermore, titanium has a low elastic modulus and, as a consequence, a titanium plate provides greater load sharing with the bone during weight-bearing. Stainless steel plates are more rigid and have less load sharing between the implant and the bone than titanium plates. Titanium plates, however, are more expensive and have more of a tendency for abrasion than stainless steel plates.

120

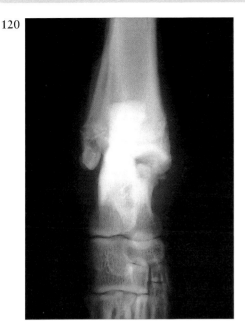

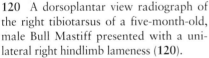

121

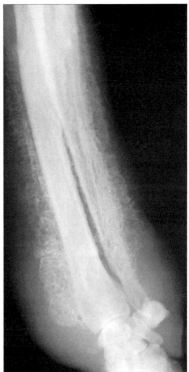

120 A dorsoplantar view radiograph of the right tibiotarsus of a five-month-old, male Bull Mastiff presented with a unilateral right hindlimb lameness (**120**).
i. What condition is affecting this dog and producing lameness?
ii. What radiograph view is most helpful for diagnosing this condition?
iii. What is the anatomic distribution of lesions in this joint?
iv. What is the recommended treatment and prognosis for this condition?

121 An eight-year-old, female Brittany Spaniel was evaluated because of swelling and lameness in all four limbs. The distal limb swelling was warm, firm and painful on deep palpation. All four limbs were equally affected. A lateral view radiograph of the dog's right antebrachium is shown (**121**). The left radius and ulna and both tibias had similar abnormalities.
i. What is the diagnosis?
ii. What other diagnostic tests should be performed to further evaluate this dog?

120 i. An OCD lesion involving the medial trochlear ridge of the talus. Typically, juvenile large breed dogs are most often affected with OCD of the talus. Clinical signs may be apparent as early as four months of age. Labrador Retrievers, Rottweilers and Bull Mastiffs are over-represented. Unlike osteochondrosis/OCD involving other sites, female dogs may be more susceptible than male dogs to developing osteochondrosis/OCD of the talus.
ii. Following localization of the lameness to the talocural joint, radiographic confirmation of the diagnosis of osteochondrosis/OCD of the talus can be difficult and requires excellent technique and often additional oblique views. The dorsal 45° medial plantarolateral oblique projection profiles the medial trochlear ridge, the dorsal 45° lateral plantaromedial oblique projection profiles the lateral trochlear ridge, and the dorsoplantar view with the talocrural joint in 10–15° flexion avoids superimposition of the calcaneus over the lateral trochlear ridge.
iii. 75% of cases affect the medial trochlear ridge and 25% of cases affect the lateral trochlear ridge. Lesions can occur anywhere along either trochlear ridge, but the plantar portion of the medial trochlear ridge is most commonly affected. Osteochondrosis/OCD of the talus is often bilateral (44%), but rarely are other joints affected simultaneously.
iv. Although the efficacy is somewhat debatable, most clinicians prefer surgical excision of the cartilage flap or osteochondral fragment. Dorsomedial, plantaromedial, dorsolateral and plantarolateral surgical approaches have been described which limit morbidity. Progression of degenerative joint disease following surgery is expected, as is some residual lameness.

121 i. Hypertrophic osteopathy or HO. This disease has also been called hypertrophic pulmonary osteopathy and hypertrophic pulmonary osteoarthropathy because of its frequent association with pulmonary disease. HO is a secondary disease found in association with chronic pulmonary diseases such as primary or secondary lung neoplasia, chronic bronchopneumonia or pulmonary abscess, and dirofilariasis. The disease has also been reported in dogs with bladder neoplasia and with hepatic adenocarcinoma.
ii. Radiographs of the thorax should be obtained to search for the primary disease responsible for the HO. If the thorax is normal, radiographic or ultrasound examinations of the abdomen should be obtained. The thoracic radiographs of this dog (see **122a, b**) revealed a primary lung neoplasm in the right caudal lobe and dirofilariasis.

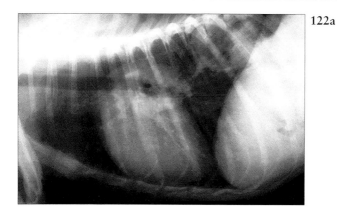

122a

122 Thoracic radiographs of the Brittany
Spaniel in 121 (122a, b). Discuss the purported
pathophysiology of HO.

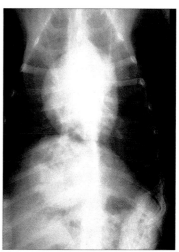

122b

123 A photograph of two bone screws of
similar length (4.0 mm cancellous screw (left)
and 3.5 mm cortical screw (right)) (123a).
i. How do these orthopedic screws differ with
regard to thread diameter, core diameter and
thread pitch?
ii. Why are these screws designed differently and
how does their design affect their application?
iii. What is the purpose of tapping during screw
application?

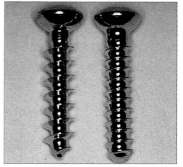

123a

122 Two theories have been proposed: the humoral theory and the neuronal theory. Neither theory is universally accepted and neither has been fully substantiated. The humoral theory suggests that thoracic diseases cause an opening of arteriovenous shunts in the lung that permit the release of vasoactive substances into the arterial circulation. These vasoactive substances, normally destroyed by the lung, cause increased peripheral blood flow in the limbs resulting in HO. Peripheral vasodilation has been experimentally induced with arteiovenous shunts, but HO has not been produced. The neuronal theory suggests that neural reflexes produced within thoracic tumors stimulate afferent fibers of the vagus nerve that subsequently stimulate efferent fibers of the distal limbs resulting in increased blood flow and the production of HO. The origin of these neural reflexes is open to question, but HO has been induced by stimulation of afferent nerve fibers believed to originate in the pulmonary hilus, mediastinum and parietal pleura. Additionally, HO will resolve when the vagus nerve is severed near the pulmonary hilus. HO also quickly regresses with appropriate treatment of the primary disease.

123 i. The 3.5 mm cortical screw has a 2.4 mm core diameter, a 3.5 mm thread diameter (0.55 mm thread height) and a 1.25 mm pitch; the 4.0 mm cancellous screw has a 1.9 mm core diameter, a 4.0 mm thread diameter (1.05 mm thread height) and a 1.75 mm thread pitch. Hence, cancellous screws have deeper, more widely spaced threads (6 threads/cm for the cancellous screw versus 8 threads/cm for the cortical screw) which provide a larger area of thread–bone contact for enhanced holding in a structurally weaker material, such as cancellous and immature bone (**123b**).

ii. Cancellous screws are available as fully and partially-threaded screws. Partially-threaded screws can be used in lag fashion without overdrilling of the *cis*-segment. Removal of partially-threaded screws can be difficult following bony ingrowth. Cortical screws are designed for use in structurally stronger materials such as dense, mature cortical bone. They have a relatively thicker core diameter and the thread design is engineered to provide maximum pullout strength in cortical bone, making them less likely to fail under shear forces as applied in plate fixation. Cortical screws are fully threaded which facilitates screw removal. These properties make cortical screws the most common choice in plate fixation.

iii. Both of these screws are designed to be inserted after the drill hole has been tapped. The tap cuts a clean and precise thread in the bone and removes debris. Tapped holes provide a more precise fit for the orthopedic screw resulting in screw placement with less torque, easier removal and reinsertion with less chance of mechanically damaging the screw hole. In softer cancellous bone, pre-tapping the screw holes may provide little or no mechanical advantage.

124 Ventrodorsal view radiograph of the pelvis of a ten-month-old, male West Highland White Terrier that has a non-weight-bearing lameness of the left hind-limb (124).
i. Describe the radiographic abnormalities.
ii. Discuss the pathologic changes that occur with this condition.
iii. What would be the most appropriate treatment for this dog?

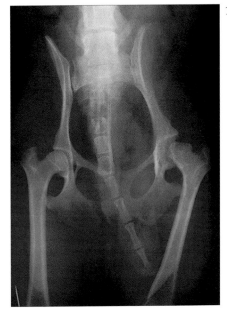

124

125 A follow-up lateral view radiograph of the right forelimb of a dog that had undergone repair of a humeral condylar fracture eight weeks previously (125).
i. Describe the complication that has occurred.
ii. List alternative methods of stabilization that may have prevented this complication.

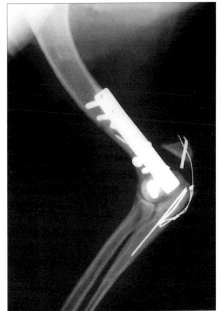

125

124 **i.** The normal trabecular pattern in the femoral neck region has been replaced by patches of increased radiodensity surrounded by areas of increased radiolucency. There is flattening of the articular surface of the femoral head, coxofemoral incongruity, and degenerative joint disease manifested by sclerosis of the subchondral bone in the region of the dorsal acetabular rim and increased radiodensity of the region of the acetabular fossa. These findings are consistent with avascular necrosis of the femoral head and secondary degenerative joint disease.

ii. The etiology of this condition has not been determined. Conjecture has centered on disruption of either the arterial or venous intraosseous and subsynovial blood flow of the femoral head and neck. Osteonecrosis occurs with ensuing trabecular resorption, fibroplasia and attempts at revascularisation. Trabecular weakness leads to subchondral bone collapse, formation of clefts and fissures in the articular cartilage, and structural deformation of the femoral head resulting in joint incongruity. Secondary generalized degenerative changes of the acetabulum also develop.

iii. Femoral head and neck excision is indicated for dogs with pain, lameness, and structural deformity of the femoral head and affords good limb function in approximately 75% of cases. Management of the dogs during the post-operative convalescent period is critical for a successful outcome as recovery is often prolonged. Attention should be given to the use of post-operative analgesia and anti-inflammatory drugs. Physiotherapy, consisting of passive flexion and extension of the coxofemoral joint, slow walks on a leash and swimming, is also critical to achieving good limb function.

125 **i.** Implant failure and resultant non-union of an olecranon osteotomy.

ii. Because of the thin profile of the canine olecranon and the narrow osteotomy bed, stabilization of olecranon osteotomies can pose a surgical challenge. Several acceptable methods for olecranon osteotomy stabilization have been described. The most common involves placement of two interfragmentary Kirschner wires and a figure-of-eight wire to form a tension band. In one retrospective study, 6 of 16 (38%) osteotomies repaired with tension band wires required a second surgery for implant removal or revision. Inaccurate implant placement accounted for the majority of failures but delayed union/non-union and fracture of the osteotomized bone were also reported. A single cancellous screw may be used, but owing to the pull of the triceps muscles at a right-angle to the longitudinal axis of the screw, cyclic failure of the screw can occur. A screw and figure-of-eight wire can be used to avoid this complication. The combined tension band and lag screw technique has been shown to provide a rapid and reliable method of fixation of olecranon osteotomies in dogs.

Plate fixation may also be utilized to stabilize olecranon osteotomies. An *in vitro* study comparing five techniques for repair of olecranon osteotomies (tension band wiring with one knot, tension band wiring with two knots, five-hole tubular plate, single screw and washer, screw and washer plus tension wiring with one knot) in human cadaveric bone found that tubular plates and tension band wiring with two knots provided the greatest stability in oblique osteotomies. Comminuted osteotomies were most rigidly stabilized by tubular plate fixation.

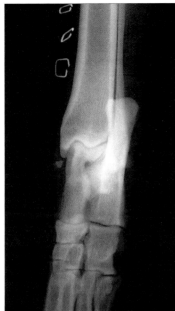

126a

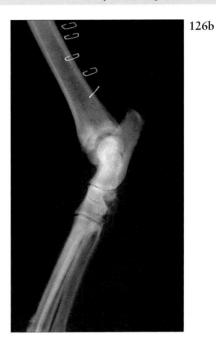

126b

126 Dorsoplantar (126a) and lateral (126b) view radiographs of the distal left hind-limb of a three-year-old, female Labrador Retriever that sustained an injury to the hock when the dog was hit by a car. The dog had a laceration over the medial aspect of the distal tibia which was debrided and closed with staples at an emergency clinic. The left talocrural joint was grossly unstable on palpation when the joint was stressed in valgus.
i. Describe the radiographic abnormalities.
ii. How should this injury be treated?

127 Name this instrument (127).

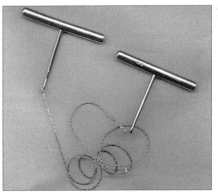

127

126c 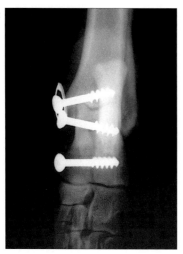 126d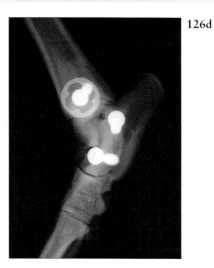

126 i. There is an avulsion fracture of the medial malleolus of the distal tibia. This fracture, along with the valgus instability elicited on palpation of the talocrural joint, infers that there is ligamentous damage. Stress view radiographs should have been performed to establish definitively the location and direction of the instability.

ii. Ligamentous support to the medial aspect of the talocrural joint must be re-established. The three major ligaments that provide stability to the medial side of the talocrural articulation are the long medial ligament and the tibiocentral and tibiotalar short component ligaments. All three ligamentous structures were damaged in this dog. Although it has been suggested that a single prosthetic ligament can be placed on the unstable side of the talocrural joint which does not tighten, loosen or shift during flexion or extension of the joint, clinical results with this technique have been less than optimal. Superior clinical results have been achieved with the placement of two prosthetic ligaments which mimic the ligaments that have been damaged. The landmarks for ligament placement on the medial aspect of the talocrural joint are the medial malleolus of the tibia (the origin of all three ligaments), the proximoplantar aspect of the talar facies (insertion of the short tibiotalar component) and the tubercle on the plantar aspect of the digital talus (insertion of the short tibiocentral ligament and the proximal insertion of the long collateral ligament). In this dog, screws were placed at these sites to anchor the prostheses. A spiked washer was used with the screw in the tibia (**126c, d**). Large diameter non-absorbable suture material was placed around at the screws in a figure-of-eight pattern. The limb was supported in a cast for three weeks following surgery and the dog was gradually returned to normal activity over the subsequent three weeks.

127 A Gigli wire bone saw with handles used to perform osteotomies.

128 A two-year-old, female German
Shorthaired Pointer developed an acute
non-weight-bearing left hindlimb lameness when the dog was hit by a slow-
moving vehicle. Radiographs revealed a
closed, diaphyseal, minimally displaced
tibial fracture. The fibula was intact. An
external coaptation device was applied to
the limb (128).
i. What is the name of this coaptation
device?
ii. What are the indications for this coaptation device's usage?
iii. What are the contraindications for this
coaptation device's usage?

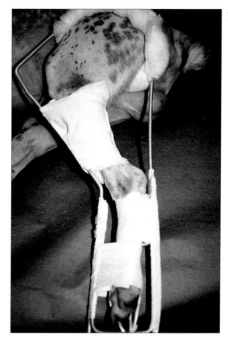

128

129 Craniocaudal (129a)
and lateral (129b) view
radiographs of the right
femur of a two-year-old
Spitz. The dog had a fracture of the right femur
eight months ago which
was initially managed by
open reduction and in-
ternal fixation using a
single intramedullary pin.
The pin was removed five
weeks following surgery
and the dog has had a
weight-bearing lameness
ever since.
i. Describe the radio-
graphic appearance of the fracture.
ii. How would this fracture be classified according to the classification scheme proposed
by Weber and Cech?

129a

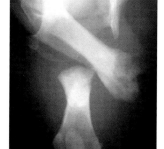

129b

128, 129: Answers

128 i. A Schroeder–Thomas splint.
ii. Schroeder–Thomas splints can be used for primary stabilization of selected fractures of the radius and ulna, and tibia and fibula. The Schroeder–Thomas splint is the only coaptation device that can be used as a traction splint. Depending on how the limb is wrapped in the splint, a Schroeder–Thomas splint can also be used to manipulate fracture segments. While Schroeder–Thomas splints were at one time used commonly in dogs and cats, their use has been largely supplanted by other treatment modalities.
iii. The cardinal rule of coaptation is that the joint proximal and distal to the injury must be immobilized. A Schroeder–Thomas splint should only be used to stabilize injuries distal to the elbow or stifle, because the splint does not adequately immobilize the scapulohumeral or coxofemoral joints.

129 i. There is a transverse mid-diaphyseal non-union fracture of the right femur with proximal and lateral displacement and angulation of the fracture segments. Bony sclerosis and exuberant callus formation are present at the ends of the fracture segments.
ii. This dog's fracture would be classified as a biologically active, hypertrophic non-union fracture. The Weber and Cech classification scheme for non-union fractures (see below) is widely used in veterinary and human orthopedics:

Biologically active (viable) non-union:
A. Hypertrophic ('elephant's foot') – prolific callus formation at the the fracture site. Fibrocartilage persists within the fracture gap as a result of continued motion.
B. Slightly hypertrophic ('horse's hoof') – callus response is minimal and there is a slight increase in the density of the ends of the fracture segments.
C. Oligotrophic – no visible callus. The ends of the fracture segments round off and there is gradual bone resorption. Evidence of remodeling is seen on serial radiographs, differentiating this viable non-union from a non-viable non-union.

Biologically inactive (non-viable) non-union:
A. Dystrophic – an intermediate fragment unites with one main fracture segment but due to compromised vascularity, fails to unite with the other main fracture segment.
B. Necrotic – intermediate necrotic fragments are present and fail to unite with the main fracture segment. The necrotic fragments appear relatively opaque on radiographs.
C. Defect – a large defect in the fracture is present; the ends of the main fracture segments usually remain viable but the area within the defect is incapable of producing bone.
D. Atrophic – the ends of fracture segments are partially resorbed. The defect between fracture segments is filled with scar tissue, incapable of osteogenic activity.

The classification scheme is based on four factors: fracture site (diaphyseal, metaphyseal, epiphyseal), displacement of fracture fragments, presence or absence of infection, and biological activity. Biological activity is the most important of these factors. The viability and osteogenic potential is dependent on the vascularity of the ends of the fracture segments. Within the categories of biologically active and inactive non-union fractures, the amount of callus present and the presence or absence of necrotic fragments identifies the non-union subcategory.

130 Lateral view radiograph of the antebrachium and carpus of a five-year-old, spayed female Yorkshire Terrier (130). The limb was injured six months previously when the dog jumped from the owner's arms. The limb has been immobilized since that time in a Mason-meta splint.
i. How would this fracture be classified according to the Weber and Cech classification scheme described in 129?
ii. What is the underlying pathogenesis for the development of this non-union fracture?
iii. What would be the most appropriate treatment for this dog?

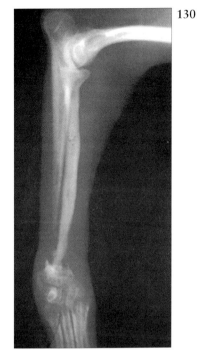

130

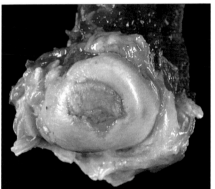

131a

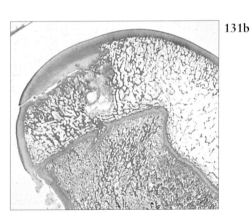

131b

131 A photograph (131a) and histologic section (131b) through the humeral head of an 11-month-old Labrador Retriever obtained at necropsy.
i. Describe the pathogenesis of this disease condition.
ii. What microscopic changes characteristic of this condition are present in the histologic section?

130 i. This fracture would be classified as a non-viable atrophic non-union of a short oblique distal diaphyseal radius and ulna fracture. Disuse osteopenia is also present.
ii. Distal radius and ulna fractures in toy breed dogs typically occur as a result of minor trauma. Although the fracture pattern is simple and the result of low energy trauma, external coaptation results in non-union in up to 85% of all such fractures. Mechanical and biological fractures have been implicated; however, the cause of the high non-union rate is not fully understood. Contraction of the carpal flexor and extensor muscles may contribute to motion at the fracture site. Coaptation of this dog in a Mason-metasplint was inappropriate as this splint does not adequately immobilize the elbow. Inadequate vascular supply has been hypothesized and recently investigated. One study found that the radial metaphyseal vasculature of small and toy breed dogs, as assessed by *ex vivo* dye injection, was subjectively less dense than that of larger breed dogs which may contribute to the high non-union rate.
iii. Successful repair would require open reduction, autogenous cancellous bone grafting, and plate fixation of the radius. Even if managed appropriately, this dog's fracture may never achieve radiographic and/or functional clinical union.

131 i. The dog has an OCD lesion of the humeral head. The humeral head is the most common site of occurrence of osteochondrosis in dogs, and lesions typically involve the central portion of the caudal aspect of the humeral head. Other concurrent pathologic abnormalities that can be seen in the gross specimen include increased thickness of the joint capsule and synovial membrane, and marginal osteophytes. Osteochondrosis is a focal disorder of endochondral ossification, including both chondrogenesis and osteo-

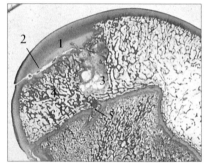

131c

genesis. Disruption of the normal process of endochondral ossification results in an increased thickness of the involved cartilage. Small fissures separating the calcified cartilage and subchondral bone develop and can become extensive enough to dissect through the cartilage to the joint surface, producing a cartilage flap as developed in this dog. This results in inflammation, lameness and the development of secondary degenerative joint disease. When this occurs the condition is more appropriately called OCD.
ii. Osteochondrosis is a focal disorder of endochondral ossification. The lesion in this specimen is confined to the caudal aspect of the humeral head (**131c**). The morphology of the remainder of the articular cartilage is normal. The articular cartilage (1) above the area of cartilage dissection (2) is thickened because endochondral ossification has been interrupted. The major alterations occur at the interface of articular cartilage with subchondral bone. The presence of subchondral bone cysts (3) and increased trabecular thickness subjacent to the lesion (4) suggest this is a chronic lesion. There is a focal fracture of the growth plate (5) suggesting that trauma may be involved in the pathogenesis of this disease.

132a
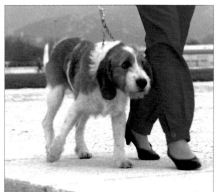

132b
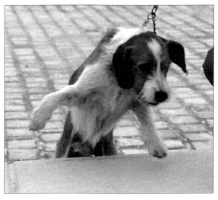

132 A photograph (132a) of a hunting dog with a chronic weight-bearing lameness of the right forelimb. The elbow is held in abduction and the antebrachium and paw are swung in a lateral arc during the swing phase of the stride. The lameness is accentuated when the dog is walked up steps (132b).
i. What is the diagnosis?
ii. What is the treatment for this condition?

133 A lateral view radiograph of the left hock of a six-year-old, male Cocker Spaniel that had undergone a talocrural arthrodesis six months previously (133). The dog had been placing increasing weight on the limb, but has developed an intermittent non-weight-bearing left hindlimb lameness over the past week.
i. Describe the complication(s) that has occurred.
ii. Why do complications occur frequently following talocrural arthrodesis?

133
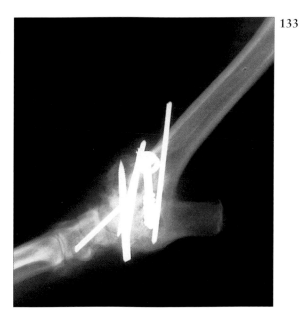

132 i. The lameness is characteristic of contracture of the infraspinatus muscle, a disabling condition that primarily affects hunting and working dogs. The condition is probably the result of trauma, but the exact etiology is unknown. Affected dogs usually have a history of acute lameness and swelling in the shoulder region associated with strenuous activity. The initial clinical signs resolve rapidly, but three to five weeks later the characteristic lameness develops and becomes progressively more severe. The infraspinatus muscle originates at the infraspinous fossa of the scapula and has its tendon of insertion on the greater tubercle of the humerus. It acts mainly to abduct and externally rotate the shoulder. As the muscle undergoes progressive fibrosis and contracture, a mechanical lameness develops with limited extension and results in persistent external rotation and abduction of the humerus. The characteristic circumduction movement of the affected limb can be accentuated if the dog is forced to walk up stairs.
ii. The lameness can be resolved by performing a tenotomy of the infraspinatus muscle. The tendon should be approached between the acromial and spinous heads of the deltoid muscle. All adhesions between the infraspinatus muscle and the joint capsule must be freed. This is done by sharp dissection and completed by aggressive flexion and extension of the scapulohumeral joint until a full range of motion is obtained.

133 i. Although the talocrural joint is no longer discernible and radiographic fusion is nearly complete, several of the implants appear to be loose. The bone screw is backing out and is no longer in direct contact with the washer. There are radiolucent zones surrounding the screw and at least two of the Steinmann pins.
ii. Several retrospective clinical studies have documented a high rate of complications associated with talocrural arthrodesis in dogs. Complications included screw fracture, implant loosening, infection and degenerative joint disease of the intertarsal and tarsometatarsal joints. The angulation of the talocrural articulation subjects implants to complex bending forces. In addition, implants are usually placed on the cranial surface of the articulation and are subjected to compressive rather than tensile forces.

In this dog the screw was placed in lag fashion to compress the arthrodesis site. The Steinmann pins were placed as adjunctive fixation to counteract rotational and bending forces. The limb was also placed in a cast for eight weeks following surgery. Failure of fixation as has occurred in this dog is common following talocrural arthrodesis. Poor owner compliance may be a factor in some cases; however, most implant complications have been attributed to inadequate fixation. Implants can only withstand loading for a finite period of time. Arthrodesis must be achieved as quickly as possible to reduce stress on the implants. Cancellous bone grafting accelerates union, thereby decreasing stress on the implants. Micromotion and chronic stresses can persist even after union and probably caused late screw loosening in this dog.

This dog's lameness resolved following implant removal. Although most dogs eventually achieve acceptable limb function following talocrural arthrodesis, lameness associated with vigorous activity is not uncommon. Pantarsal arthrodesis, stabilized with a bone plate, results in satisfactory limb function with a lower incidence of complications and would appear to be a better treatment for dogs with severe instability or degeneration of the talocrural joint.

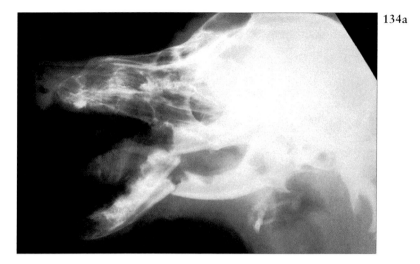

134a

134 A lateral view radiograph of the skull of a 12-year-old, female Poodle with severe, generalized periodontal disease (134a). During a routine prophylactic dental cleaning an audible crack was heard during extraction of both mandibular first molars.
i. Describe the radiographic abnormalities.
ii. Give two treatment plans and discuss the rationale for each approach.

135 A two-year-old, spayed female Labrador Retriever was presented with a three-month history of right hindlimb lameness. On physical examination crepitus could be elicited from the right stifle. Under sedation, 3–5 mm of cranial drawer motion could be elicited. Radiographs of the right stifle revealed a synovial effusion and moderate degenerative changes. Synovial fluid was collected from the affected stifle. The nucleated cell count was 4.5×10^9 cells/l and the viscosity was normal.

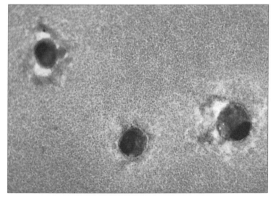

135

i. What are the landmarks for arthrocentesis of the stifle?
ii. Give a cytologic description and interpretation of the lesion (135).

134 i. All the teeth are absent. There is marked resorption of the alveolar bone and the rostral mandible. There is remodeling and attrition of the rostral maxilla and mandible. There is a pathologic fracture of both horizontal ramus of both mandibles.

134b

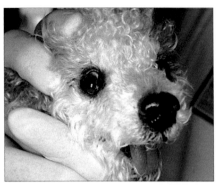

ii. The fractures could be stabilized using an external skeletal fixator, an intraoral splint or bone plates and screws. Obtaining bone union in a dog such as this with extensive periodontal disease is difficult due to age-related prolonged healing times, pre-existing bone loss and contamination or infection at the fracture sites. In addition, obtaining adequate purchase of the mandible with fixation pins or screws may be difficult because of the poor quality of the mandibular bone. Implant loosening following surgery would also be a concern. Attempts to stabilize the fractures in this dog has the potential for multiple reparative procedures which might result in fibrous union at best.

Rostral mandibulectomy is a reasonable treatment alternative for older dogs with few or no remaining teeth and extensive periodontal disease. Most dogs undergoing rostral mandibulectomy for neoplastic disease have acceptable masticatory function and cosmetic appearance following surgery. In this dog, rostral mandibulectomy was performed as a definitive salvage procedure and yielded a good clinical outcome (**134b**). The chin and ventral lip required soft tissue reconstruction following resection of the rostral mandible. The procedure involved removal of a full-thickness triangle of skin. The base of the triangle was positioned rostrally. The most critical suture is the first suture placed at the mucocutaneous junction. The remaining defect is apposed in three layers to approximate the soft tissues near the mandibular resection/fracture sites.

135 i. The approach is typically from the craniolateral aspect of the stifle. With the joint slightly flexed, the entry point is located just lateral to the patellar ligament, midway between the proximal aspect of the patella and the tibial tuberosity. The needle is directed caudomedially toward the intercondylar space.

ii. The background is dense, granular and eosinophilic, indicating a normal mucin content. The nucleated cells present are all macrophages. These cells are reactive as demonstrated by increased cytoplasmic vacuolation and basophilia. The interpretation would be non-inflammatory joint fluid consistent with degenerative joint disease. Normal synovial fluid in dogs should contain less than 3×10^9 nucleated cells/l, the vast majority of which (>90%) should be mononuclear cells (lymphocytes, monocytes, macrophages and a few synovial lining cells). A mild elevation in nucleated cell counts, with a significant population of reactive macrophages, is typical of synovial fluid seen with degenerative joint diseases.

136 With regard to the Labrador Retriever in **135**, discuss possible etiologies.

137 A schematic drawing of a dog's femur which has a mid-diaphyseal fracture (**137a**).
i. What type of loading caused the spiral fracture shown?
ii. What type of stresses are present along the fracture plane in a bone loaded to create a spiral fracture?

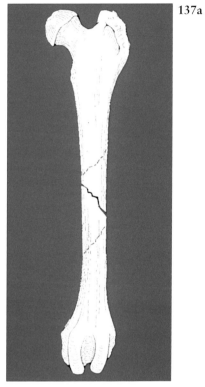

137a

138 Name this surgical instrument (**138**).

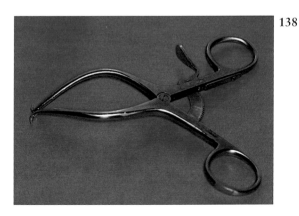

138

136 Any number of conditions may precipitate the development of degenerative joint disease. Traumatic osteochondral or ligamentous injuries and developmental joint abnormalities are potential etiologies. This dog's stifle was explored and at surgery a partial tear of the CCL was found.

137 i. Torsional loading (137b, large arrows).

ii. Torsional loading of a bone generates maximum shear stresses on the outer surface of the bone which serve as the initial site of fracture propagation in spiral fractures. After the fracture initiates on the surface of the bone, it propagates along the plane of maximum tensile stress (small arrows), which is oblique to the spiral plane along the length of the bone. Forces can be applied to structures in various directions, producing tension, compression, bending, shear and torsion. In addition, any or all of these forces can be applied simultaneously producing combined loading. Under *tensile loading*, the plane of maximum stress is perpendicular to the applied load. As the structure is pulled in tension, it lengthens and narrows. Microscopically, the structure fails by debonding of the cement lines, and the structure fails transversely. The bones most commonly fractured clinically by tensile forces are the olecranon and the calcaneus. In *compression* the plane of maximum compressive stress is perpendicular to the applied load. Under compressive loading, the structure shortens and widens. The plane of maximum shear stress in a structure loaded in compression is at 45° to the applied load. Microscopically, the structure fails by oblique cracking of the osteons in a 45° plane to the long axis of the bone along the plane of maximum shear. Vertebral body fractures are often pro-

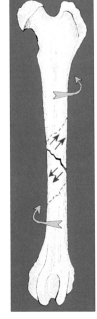

137b

duced by compression forces. *Bending* causes a structure to bend around an axis with the result that the structure is subjected to both compressive and tensile forces, simultaneously. Tensile stresses act on one side of the neutral axis and compressive stresses on the opposite side. No stresses act at the neutral axis. The magnitude of the stresses are proportional to their distance from the neutral axis. The farther from the neutral axis, the higher the stresses. Fractures that are produced by bending typically begin with a transverse fracture initiated on the surface subjected to tension, which then traverses across the diaphysis of the bone before diverging into a butterfly fragment. The initial transverse portion of the fracture fails along the line of maximum tensile stress and the arms of the butterfly fragment fail along the lines of maximum shear stress. When a structure is subjected to *shear*, the load is applied parallel to the surface of the structure. A structure subjected to shear stresses deforms in an angular manner; right angles on the surface of the structure become more acute. Shear fractures are most commonly seen in regions containing cancellous bone. Fractures of the humeral condyle and the tibial plateau are examples.

138 Gelpi retractors.

139a

139 Lateral (139a) and cranio-caudal (139b) view radiographs of a comminuted femur fracture stabilized with a bone plate.
i. What type of plate was used to stabilize this fracture?
ii. What was the intended application of this type of plate?
iii. List two advantageous properties of this type of plate.
iv. What is the major disadvantage of this type of plate?

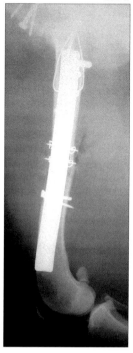

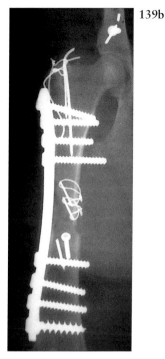

139b

140 A six-month-old, male Rottweiler is presented with a five-day history of an acute onset with consistent weight-bearing right forelimb lameness which worsens with exercise. Physical evaluation reveals thickening of the metacarpophalangeal joint of the second digit of the right forepaw. Flexion of this joint is reduced and elicits a marked pain response. A dorsopalmar view radiograph of the right forepaw is shown (**140**).
i. Describe the radiographic abnormalities.
ii. What clinical data are helpful in determining whether the lesion(s) present on this radiograph is/are the cause of this dog's lameness?

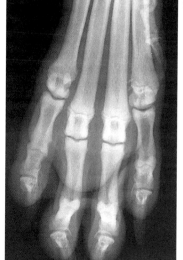

140

139 i.
A 4.5 mm narrow lengthening plate (**139c**, top). A 4.5 mm broad lengthening plate (**139c**, bottom) is also available which can be identified by the serpentine pattern of the screw hole position.

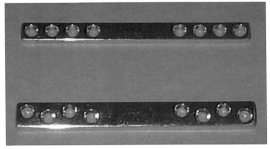

139c

ii. Lengthening plates were devised for lengthening tibial osteotomies in humans; however, these plates are often used in dogs in a buttress application to bridge a bony region with little or no structural strength such as severely comminuted diaphyseal fractures.

iii. In complicated, comminuted fractures in which the fracture site is unlikely to contribute substantially to the transfer of load during weight-bearing, the plate must essentially support all of the forces transmitted through the limb. This requires a very rigid, strong plate–bone construction. When an open hole in the plate is positioned over a bony defect, which is often impossible to avoid in severely comminuted fractures stabilized with conventional plates, the stress generated within the plate is increased 14 times. In addition, DCPs have oval screw holes to provide bone–plate displacement used for compression, but when used in a buttress mode, oval holes allow undesirable shifting and minor motion between the bone and plate. Lengthening plates are devoid of central screw holes and have round screw holes which closely conform to the shape of the screw heads, thus maximizing screw-plate stability.

iv. The lack of holes in the central portion of the plate does not allow central fracture segments to be rigidly stabilized to the plate.

140 i.
The second and seventh palmar metacarpal sesamoid bones are fragmented. The proximal pole of the second palmar metacarpal sesamoid bone is disrupted into three fragments, with two of the fragments displaced proximally and laterally. The seventh palmar metacarpal sesamoid bone appears to have increased lucency centrally, and the proximal pole of this sesamoid is displaced proximally, indicating possible disruption of this sesamoid as well.

ii. The thickening and reduced range of flexion of the second metacarpophalangeal joint are probably due to the disruption of the second sesamoid bone. The pain response on flexion of the second metacarpophalangeal joint suggests the lameness is associated with the abnormalities present in this joint. The absence of physical examination abnormalities associated with the fifth metacarpophalangeal joint suggests that the radiographic lesion in the seventh sesamoid is of no clinical importance. The remainder of the limb should also be examined to eliminate alternative causes of the lameness.

141 With regard to the Rottweiler in 140, what treatment should be recommended?

142 Immediate (142a, b) and 12 months post-operative (142c, d) radiographs from a neutered male Springer Spaniel which underwent a cementless total hip replacement at 13 months of age. A parital osteotomy of the greater trochanter at the insertion of the deep gluteal tendon was performed to improve exposure and was replaced and stabilized using a single cerclage wire.
i. Describe the radiographic appearance of the 12 months' post-operative films compared with the initial films.
ii. What are the possible causes responsible for the radiographic changes?

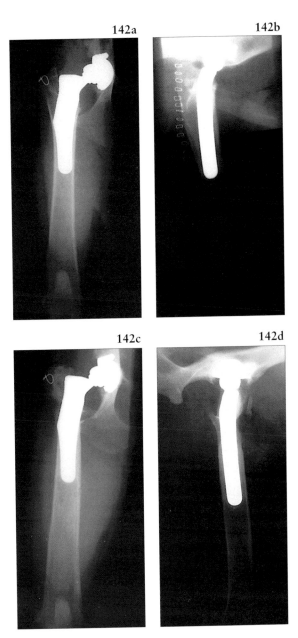

142a 142b

142c 142d

141 The dog should be confined and only allowed short walks while on a lead for four to six weeks. The lameness associated with fragmentation of the palmar metacarpal sesamoid bones is transient in the vast majority of affected dogs. If the lameness does not improve and no other cause of lameness is found, excision of the second sesamoid bone is indicated. The bone is approached through a palmar incision, incising the superficial digital flexor tendon and displacing the deep digital flexor tendon laterally. The intersesamoidean ligament and the other sesamoidean ligaments are sharply incised close to the bone and the fragmented sesamoid bone is removed. The superficial digital flexor tendon is sutured with 4-0 absorbable suture and the other layers are closed routinely. A firm, well-padded bandage is applied for two weeks following surgery, after which a gradual return to normal activity is permitted.

142 i. The 12-month post-operative radiographs show resorption of the proximomedial (calcar region), lateral, cranial and caudal femoral cortices. The femoral cortices distal to the implant elbow (lateral flare) are hypertrophied. There is a bone fragment cranial to the femur which represents a non-union of the greater trochanteric osteotomy.
ii. Bone resorption of the proximal portion of the femur has been attributed to stress shielding, vascular injury from reaming and implantation of femoral stems and reaction to wear debris. Stress shielding occurs with all femoral stems whether cemented or cementless. The altered stresses result in bone resorption which is commonly observed radiographically in the calcar region, but can occur in other areas. Resorption, if severe enough, may result in avulsion fractures of the lesser and greater trochanters, and loosening of the prosthesis. Stress shielding is strongly influenced by the load transfer mechanism and implant stiffness. The level of the load transfer is influenced by the extent of porous coating, collar–calcar contact and interface stability. Distal load transfer may occur by bone ingrowth occurring distally into a fully coated stem or achieving a tight distal fit with a wedge-shaped stem. A collar will increase the load transfer proximally through the calcar, and therefore decrease the probability of developing stress shielding. Femoral stems made of materials with a lower modulus of elasticity, such as titanium, will decrease stress shielding.

Medullary reaming and femoral stem implantation results in increased metaphyseal porosity, vascularity and bone formation which contribute to remodeling of the proximal portion of the femur. Polyethylene and metal wear debris from articulating surfaces and interfaces of titanium and cobalt stems induce osteolysis through activation of collagenase, macrophages and osteoclasts and through mechanical factors. Loose total hip components produce a larger volume of wear debris compared with stable implants.

143 A necropsy specimen of a dog's stifle which has been disarticulated (143a). The caudal pole of the medial meniscus has been crushed and is fibrillated (circled).
i. How can the medial meniscus be evaluated at arthrotomy?
ii. What would be the appropriate treatment for a medial meniscal lesion such as the one illustrated?

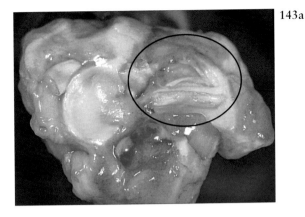

143a

144 A photograph of the right hindlimb of a two-year-old female Bulldog that had a pantarsal arthrodesis performed two months previously which was stabilized with a transarticular circular fixator (144). What four surgical principles are considered essential to perform an arthrodesis?

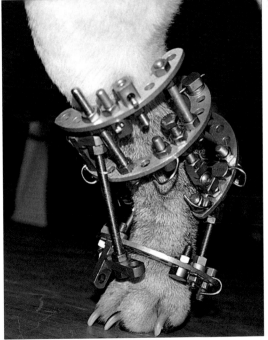

144

143 i. More than 90% of meniscal pathology involves the caudal pole of the medial meniscus. Unfortunately, the caudal pole of the medial meniscus is difficult to visualize. The following techniques assist in exposing the medial meniscus: (1) Use of lavage-suction to clear synovial fluid or blood from the joint. (2) Use of a Senn retractor to elevate the joint capsule and pull the tibia into cranial drawer. (3) Insertion of a Hohmann retractor into the intercondylar notch, positioning the tip of the retractor over the caudal aspect of the tibial plateau. The retractor can be levered

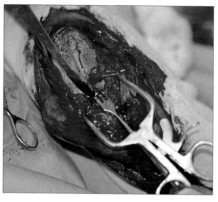

against the femoral trochlea to push the tibia cranially and away from the femoral condyles. A Gelpi retractor is also being used to facilitate visualization in this photograph (143b).

The caudal pole of a normal medial meniscus may fold forward if cranial drawer is present. This can mimic a meniscal tear. The meniscus should be pushed back into normal position and re-evaluated. The meniscus should be left intact or *in situ* unless damaged and the joint stabilized by an appropriate technique.

ii. The damaged meniscal tissue should be excised. Complete meniscectomy induces degenerative joint disease by altering load distribution and transmission through the joint. Therefore, alternatives to total meniscectomy should be considered where appropriate. Caudal pole hemimeniscectomy conferred no significant advantage over total medial meniscectomy in one experimental study in sheep but has been used in dogs. If a single longitudinal midsubstance tear of the caudal pole is found, the detached axial portion of the meniscus (the 'bucket handle') should be excised and the outer rim of meniscus preserved. Preservation of one-third or more of the outer rim retains much of the biomechanical functions of the meniscus.

The menisci are composed of avascular fibrocartilage. Midsubstance tears of the meniscus will only heal if the lesion communicates with the vascular synovial attachments at the meniscus' periphery. A full-thickness radial incision in the meniscus (vascular access channel) may allow the tear in the meniscus to regenerate. Such an incision, however, impairs the function of the circumferentially orientated collagen fibers in transmitting load through the meniscus and is not recommended.

144 (1) Removal of all articular cartilage from the joint surfaces involved in the arthrodesis. (2) Implantation of a cancellous bone graft in the former joint space to accelerate bone union. (3) Application of rigid internal and/or external fixation with compression of the joint surfaces when possible. (4) Placement of the involved limb segment in a functional anatomic position.

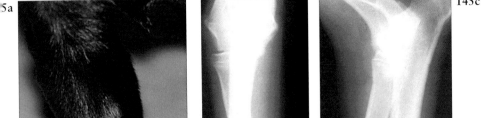
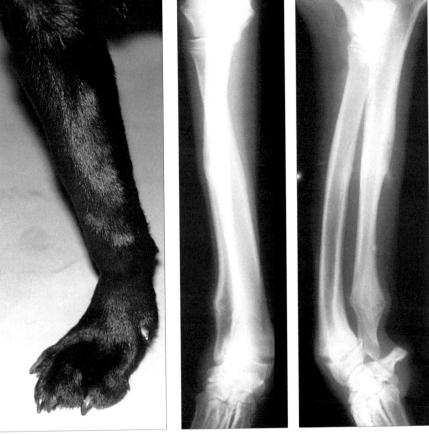

145 A photograph of the right forelimb of a ten-month-old, male Labrador Retriever presenting with a right forelimb lameness (145a). Craniocaudal (145b) and lateral (145c) view radiographs of the right antebrachium are shown.
i. What is the diagnosis?
ii. What is the percentage of total long bone growth contributed by the proximal radial physis, the distal radial physis, the proximal ulnar physis and the distal ulnar physis?
iii. Why is the distal ulnar physis predisposed to premature closure?
iv. Describe how an oblique corrective osteotomy and stabilization with a type II external fixator would be performed to correct this dog's deformity.

146 What are the components of the Achilles tendon?

145 i. Premature closure of the distal ulnar physis resulting in shortening and cranial bowing of the radius with valgus angulation and external rotation of the carpus.
ii. Proximal radial physis – 40%; distal radial physis – 60%; to the length of the radius. Proximal ulnar physis – 15%; distal ulnar physis – 85%; to the length of the ulna.
iii. The conical shape of the distal ulnar physis predisposes the physis to Salter–Harris type V fractures resulting in premature physeal closure.
iv. The proximal and distal transfixation pins are placed in the metaphyses. The pins should parallel their respective proximal and distal radial articular surfaces and be within the lateral transverse plane of each segment. Centrally-threaded positive profile fixation pins should be used.

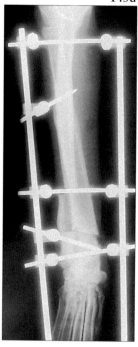
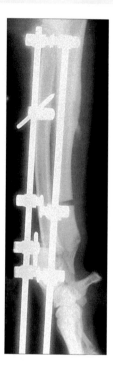

A transverse ulnar osteotomy is performed with an osteotome or oscillating saw. An oblique osteotomy of the radius is made at the point of greatest curvature, directing the osteotomy line parallel to the distal radial articular surface. The proximal and distal transfixation pins are aligned parallel to each other and in the same transverse plane which should eliminate angular and rotational deformity. One to two additional fixation pins should be placed in each radial segment.

Post-operative radiographs are made to document radial alignment and implant position (145d, e). Correction of residual angular deformity can be made by loosening the clamps on the distal fixation pins and realigning the distal bone segment. Correction of residual rotational deformity can be made by removing one connecting rod and rotating the single clamps so that the pins in the distal segment are positioned on the opposite side of the connecting rod.

146 There are three separate components: (1) The tendon of the gastrocnemius muscle, which inserts at the tuber calcanei. (2) The superficial digital flexor tendon, which glides across the tuber calcanei and extends to the level of the middle phalanges. (3) The common tendon of the biceps femoris, semitendinosus and gracilis muscles, which inserts at the tuber calcanei.

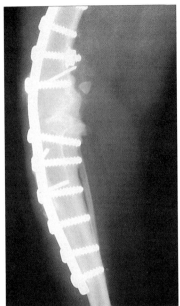
147a

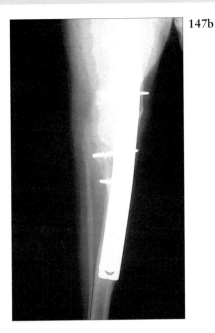
147b

147 A 12-month-old, intact male German Shepherd Dog presented with a history of a right distal femoral fracture which was stabilized with an intramedullary pin when the dog was six months old. Radiographs of the right hindlimb revealed migration of the implants from the previous fracture repair into the stifle resulting in severe degenerative joint disease. An arthrodesis of the right stifle was performed (**147a, b**).
i. What are two main factors are thought to influence limb function following stifle arthrodesis?
ii. Why was this method of internal fixation utilized for stifle arthrodesis in this large breed dog?
iii. What guideline(s) is used when considering the appropriate angle of arthrodesis for the stifle?

148 A photograph of a pair of surgical implants (**148a**).
i. Name the implants.
ii. What is the intended use for these implants?
iii. Discuss the clinical complications which have been ascribed to the use of these implants.

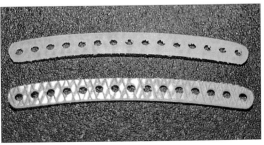
148a

147 i. The ability to effectively place the paw to the ground without a substanial change in posture of the contralateral limb and a normal range of motion in the ipsilateral coxo-femoral joint. These two factors influence the function of both the limb that has had the stifle arthrodesed as well as the contralateral hindlimb.

ii. The most appropriate form of fixation for performing a stifle arthrodesis in this case was a bone plate applied to the cranial surface of the stifle. Application of the bone plate to the cranial surface facilitates contouring of the plate and provides optimal stability as the cranial surface of the stifle is the tension surface during weight-bearing. The bone plate selected should accommodate placement of at least three screws on either side of the arthrodesis. Increasing the number of cortices engaged by screws on each side of the arthrodesis should lessen the possibility of screw loosening, as well as decrease the bending moment which is concentrated at the most proximal and distal screw holes.

iii. The normal standing angle of the contralateral stifle should be measured to determine the appropriate angle of arthrodesis. If the contralateral hindlimb is normal, 5–10° of extension should be added to the measured angle to allow for shortening caused by the procedure. In some instances the limb may not be long enough if the contralateral stifle angle is used, therefore it is advisable to error on the side of placing the joint at a slightly greater angle of extension.

148 i. Plastic spinal plates. The plates are machined from sheets of polyvinylidine fluoride. The plates were developed by two surgeons, Drs Lumb and Brasner, and are known as Lubra plates.

ii. To stabilize the vertebral column. Lubra plates were designed to be used in pairs with one plate positioned on either side of the dorsal spinous processes. Note that grooves are stamped into one surface of the plate. The roughened surfaces of the plates should be opposed, engaging the dorsal spinous processes, when the plates are applied. Wilson bolts are placed through the holes in the plates, between dorsal spinous processes, and the bolts are secured with washers and nuts. As the nuts are tightened, the plates grip the dorsal spinous processes (**148b**).

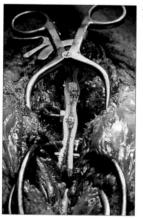

148

iii. Implant failure, specifically dorsal displacement of the plates. Proper application of the plates is critical to prevent implant failure. The plates should be placed as ventral as possible on the dorsal spinous processes. Grooving the dorsal lamina adjacent to the dorsal spinous processes and positioning the vertebral column in slight flexion so the vertebral column conforms to the curve of the plates facilitates ventral plate placement. In addition, a minimum of three dorsal spinous processes cranial and caudal to the lesion should be engaged. It has been suggested that Lubra plates cause ischemic necrosis of the dorsal spinous processes. Although loss of bone density of the dorsal spinous processes is often noted one to three months following application of Lubra plates, experimental studies have shown that plate application does not devitalize the engaged dorsal spinous processes.

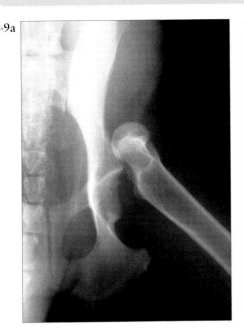

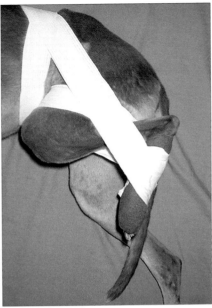

149b

149 A radiograph of a dog with a traumatic coxofemoral luxation (149a) that was reduced in a closed fashion and stabilized by external coaptation (149b).
i. The diagnosis of a coxofemoral luxation is generally made on physical examination. Why should radiographs of the coxofemoral joint be obtained?
ii. Name the type of external coaptation used to stabilize the reduction.
iii. Describe the technique of applying this type of coaptation.

150 A dog was hit by a car and became non-weight-bearing on the left forelimb. A lateral radiograph of the affected limb is shown (150).
i. What eponym is commonly associated with this injury?
ii. Outline the classification scheme used to categorize this type of injury.
iii. Briefly describe the biomechanical event which produces this type of injury.

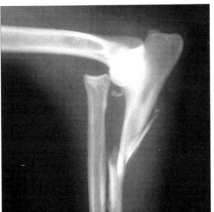

150

149 i. Radiographs should be obtained to confirm the diagnosis and to determine the direction of the luxation. Radiographs are also obtained to identify concurrent traumatic injuries such as acetabular fractures, avulsion fractures of the femoral head, fractures involving the proximal femoral physis, and femoral neck or trochanteric fractures. The radiographs should also be evaluated for the presence of pre-existing coxofemoral joint conformational abnormalities or degenerative joint disease which might indicate the presence of hip dysplasia or Legg–Calvé–Perthes disease. Concurrent traumatic fractures or developmental abnormalities may preclude attempts at closed reduction of the luxation and make surgical intervention (open reduction and stabilization, femoral head and neck excision or total hip replacement) the more appropriate treatment option.
ii. An Ehmer sling.
iii. After the luxation is reduced, a thin cast padding and gauze bandage is applied to the paw to help prevent skin necrosis. The digits are left exposed so that they can be evaluated for swelling while the sling is in place. The tarsus and stifle are flexed. Adhesive tape is placed from the lateral aspect of the metatarsus, under the medial aspect of the thigh proximal to the stifle joint, over the cranial and lateral aspects of the thigh, medial and caudal to the tarsus, and back to the lateral aspect of the metatarsus. This figure-of-eight pattern is repeated several times to maintain flexion, internal rotation and slight abduction of the femur. The sling must be positioned as proximal as possible on the thigh to prevent the adhesive tape from slipping over the stifle. Additional abduction and flexion of the coxofemoral joint is achieved by taping from the metatarsal bandage over the dog's dorsum and around the abdomen, being careful to avoid the prepuce in male dogs. The Ehmer sling prevents weight-bearing and internally rotates, flexes and abducts the femur to maximize dorsal acetabular coverage of the femoral head. Radiographs are obtained after the sling is applied to ensure the joint is still reduced. The sling is usually maintained for approximately two weeks until healing of the joint capsule and periarticular fibrosis is sufficient to maintain joint congruency.

150 i. A Monteggia lesion is an ulnar fracture with a concurrent luxation of the radial head.
ii. Bado classified Monteggia lesions into four types. Type I: diaphyseal fracture of the ulna with cranial dislocation of the radial head. This is the most common type. Type II: diaphyseal fracture of the ulna with caudal dislocation of the radial head. Type III: diaphyseal fracture of the ulna with lateral or craniolateral dislocation of the radial head. Type IV: fracture of the ulna, fracture of the proximal third of the radius and cranial dislocation of the radial head. This dog has a type I lesion.
iii. Monteggia lesions are caused by a blow to the caudal aspect of the ulna while the antebrachium is extended and weight-bearing. The blunt force causes a fracture of the ulna, with a concurrent luxation of the radial head, either the result of a rupture of the radial annular ligament or fracture of the radius.

151 With regard to the dog in 150, how should this injury be treated?

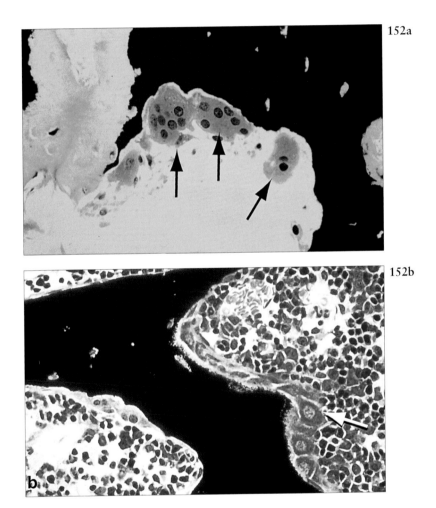

152a

152b

152 Histologic sections of cancellous bone tissue stained according to the Von Kossa method with a tetrachrome counterstain (×400) (152a, b).
i. Identify the bone cells indicated by the arrows.
ii. What are the defining characteristics of each cell type and their major function?

151 The fractured ulna should be anatomically reduced and stabilized with a plate, intramedullary pin and cerclage wires or screws placed in lag fashion. If the ulna is stabilized in a shortened position, reduction of the radial head may be difficult. Initial radial head reduction may prevent this problem. The torn radial annular ligament should be sutured if possible. If primary ligament repair is used as the sole means of radial head stabilization, there is a high incidence (32%) of reluxation of the radial head. Thus, supplemental fixation is advised. Placement of a bone screw(s) or a hemicerclage wire(s) between the proximal ulna and radius is often performed.

If a screw or wire is placed from the ulna to the radius in an immature animal, disparity in the growth of the ulna and radius can result in elbow incongruency and limb deformity. In addition, if a synostosis develops between the radius and ulna, normal pronation and supination may be limited. Screw or wire removal should be done three to five weeks following surgery to improve pronation and supination of the antebrachium.

152 i. The arrows in **152a** point to osteoclasts, and the arrow in **152b** points to an osteoblast.

ii. Osteoclasts are large, irregularly shaped, multinucleated cells, with one or two prominent nucleoli per nucleus which are responsible for bone resorption. Their acidophilic cytoplasm has a foamy appearance due to the presence of many vacuoles. Osteoclasts are always found adjacent to bone surfaces within scalloped resorption pits known as Howship's lacunae. At its interface with bone, the surface of the osteoclast appears to be striated due to the presence of a ruffled border, an area of extensive membrane infoldings that is best observed by electron microscopy. The presence of a ruffled border is essential for bone resorptive activity. Osteoclasts release lysosomal enzymes in the local microenvironment under the ruffled border to degrade bone matrix. These bone resorbing cells are responsive to several drugs and hormones. For example, parathyroid hormone stimulates osteoclastic activity, whereas estrogen, calcitonin and bisphosphonates inhibit osteoclastic activity.

Osteoblasts are the bone forming cells that synthesize and secrete bone matrix. Osteoblasts are plump, cuboidal cells with a single, eccentric nucleus. They become more flattened in appearance in aged animals. In contrast to osteoclasts, the cytoplasm of osteoblasts has basophilic staining characteristics. A prominent, pale staining Golgi apparatus is usually apparent adjacent to the nucleus. The plasma membrane of the osteoblast is rich in alkaline phosphatase. Osteoblasts are never seen singly but rather occur in groups lining bone surfaces. A layer of osteoid, or unmineralized bone matrix, is often seen between the osteoblasts and the bone surface. Osteoblasts that become sequestered in lacunae within the bone matrix are known as osteocytes. The activity of osteoblasts is influenced by many diverse factors such as age, mechanical loading, hormones and growth factors.

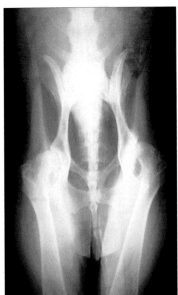

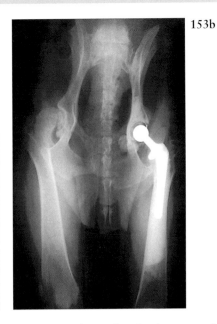

153 Pre-operative (153a) and post-operative (153b) radiographs of a four-year-old Golden Retriever with hip dysplasia who has undergone left total hip replacement.
i. What is the radiodense material anchoring the prosthesis in the bone?
ii. What is the purpose of the radiodense oval wire in the acetabular area?
iii. What is the overall reported complication rate with this procedure, and what are the most commonly reported complications?

154 A necropsy specimen obtained from a seven-month-old, male Rottweiler that had a right forelimb lameness (154a). The right elbow has been disarticulated and the ulna has been transversely sectioned through the trochlear notch. The articular surface of the proximal radius and ulna can be seen in the photograph. Describe the lesion present in this joint.

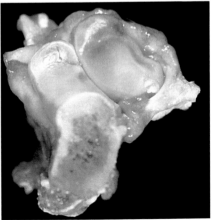

153 i. This particular prosthesis is a cemented design, which uses PMMA bone cement to anchor the prosthesis to the bone. PMMA by itself is radiolucent; however, barium is frequently added to medical grade PMMA to make it visible on radiographs (observe the post-operative radiographs). PMMA is not an adhesive, but when the liquid monomer and powdered polymer are mixed an exothermic reaction occurs and the cement mass solidifies in approximately eight to ten minutes. The cement acts very much like a grout, and implant stability depends on a physical interlock between the cement–bone interface. To this end, a number of techniques have been developed to maximize the bone-cement interface. The cement can be mixed under a vacuum or centrifuged after an initial mixing phase. This yields a biomechanically stronger cement mass. The recipient bed should be clean, dry, and free of blood. A number of cement delivery systems have been described in both the human and veterinary literature. Femoral canal restrictors, pressurized cement guns and low viscosity cement have resulted in improved cement–bone interlock and improved clinical success with cemented techniques in humans.

ii. The acetabular component is radiolucent ultra-high-molecular-weight polyethylene and cannot be visualized on the post-operative radiographs. The wire is embedded in the acetabular component and serves as a marker allowing the positioning and stability of the acetabular component to be evaluated. The wire should be placed so it appears oval shaped on both the ventrodorsal and lateral views. An estimate of the acetabular version angle can be measured on the ventrodorsal radiograph by drawing a line through the apices of the oval and measuring the angle formed between this line and a vertical line drawn through the center of the femoral head.

iii. In 1996 it was approximately 5–10%. Loosening of components is the most frequently reported complication following total hip replacement. Loosening can either be biologic (septic or aseptic) or mechanical in nature. In some instances these failures can be revised to successful outcomes. Dislocations, fractures, sciatic neuropraxia and implant related sarcomas are less commonly reported complications.

154 Fragmentation of the medial coronoid process of the ulna is present in this elbow. A curvilinear fracture line is visible in the articular surface of the lateral portion of the medial coronoid process adjacent to the radial head (**154b**, arrows). The lesion in this elbow would be more appropriately described as a fissure rather than a fragment because the involved portion of the medial coronoid process was not freely movable and, upon further dissection and histopathologic examination, the fissure did not extend fully through the subchondral bone.

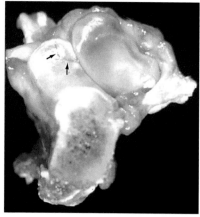

154

155 What is the etiopathogenesis of the condition affecting the Rottweiler in 154?

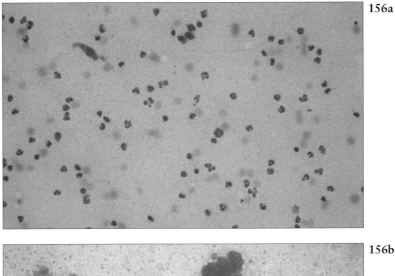

156a

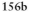

156b

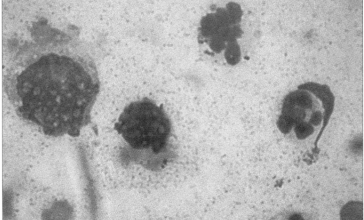

156 A ×16 (156a) and a ×100 (156b) photograph of Wright–Giemsa stained cytologic preparations of synovial fluid aspirated from the stifle joint of a five-year-old,
neutered female Old English Sheepdog.
i. Describe the cytologic features seen on these slides.
ii. What is the most likely diagnosis?
iii. What specific diagnostic technique will yield the best chance of a definitive diagnosis?
iv. What general mechanisms are responsible for the development of this condition?

155 The etiopathogenesis of fragmented coronoid process remains controversial. Fragmented coronoid process was originally believed to be a manifestation of osteochondrosis; however, pathoanatomic studies have not supported this theory. Histologically, these lesions are more consistent with traumatic osteochondral fractures in various states of attempted repair (155). Most investigators currently prescribe to the theory that fragmentation of

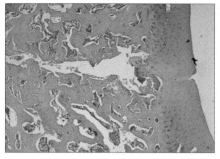

the coronoid process occurs as a consequence of elbow joint incongruity. Incongruity has been recognized in affected dogs as distal subluxation of the radial head which places the distal margin of the trochlear notch and the medial coronoid process slightly proximal to the articular surface of the radial head. This anatomic relationship places excessive loads on the developing coronoid process resulting in fragmentation. Two mechanisms, asynchronous growth of the radius and ulna and underdevelopment of the trochlear notch of the ulna, have been suggested as causes for this incongruency.

156 i. Degenerate neutrophils are present in large numbers. A few mononuclear cells and synoviocytes can also be seen. Phagocytosed cocci are present within a degenerate neutrophil and macrophage when the slide is examined under high power (×100 objective).
ii. Septic arthritis.
iii. Although the presence of large numbers of neutrophils in the synovial fluid is suggestive of septic arthritis, immune-mediated arthropathies must also be considered, particularly if neutrophils are non-degenerate. The presence of bacteria in the synovial fluid in this dog substantiates the diagnosis of septic arthritis; however, many cases of septic arthritis will not have obvious bacteria present on microscopic examination of the synovial fluid. In most cases, culture of synovial fluid is critical to a diagnosis of septic arthritis; however, approximately 50% of synovial fluid cultures from infected joints will initially yield false-negative results. Inoculating synovial fluid into blood culture medium and incubating for 24 hours (37°C/98.6°F), followed by inoculation onto blood agar, significantly increases the possibility of obtaining positive cultures. It is recommended that synovial fluid samples be inoculated onto an aerobic culturette as well as into blood culture medium. The aerobic culturette can be cultured immediately while the sample in the blood culture medium can be subcultured after 24 hours if the culturette sample has yielded no growth. Synovial fluid is as or more likely to yield positive cultures than synovial membrane samples if this protocol is followed.
iv. Joint infections can be initiated by hematogenous spread of bacterial organisms to the joint from a remote site of infection, extension of a local (juxta-articular) infection into the joint or traumatic penetration of the joint. Joints may also be infected iatrogenically as a result of articular surgery or intra-articular injections. The most common organisms isolated from infected joints in dogs and cats include *Staphylococcus* spp., *Streptococcus* spp., *Corynebacterium* spp., *Escherichia coli* and other coliforms.

157a 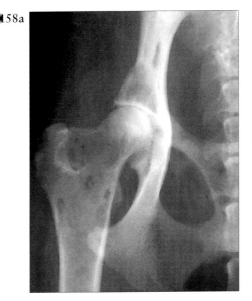 157b

157 A transverse ultrasound image of a right common calcaneal tendon in a dog presented for chronic lameness (157a). A sonogram of the contralateral normal tendon is also provided (157b).
i. What abnormalities are evident in the affected tendon?
ii. What is the diagnostic value of ultrasonography in evaluating dogs and cats suspected of having tendon injuries?

158a

158b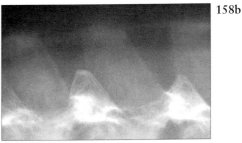

158 Ventrodorsal view radiograph (158a) of the pelvis and lateral view radiograph (158b) of the dorsal spinous processes of the lumbar vertebral column of an 11-year-old Chesapeake Bay Retriever presented for hindlimb weakness and pain.
i. Describe the radiographic abnormalities present.
ii. What is the most likely diagnosis?

157, 158: Answers

157 i. The right common calcaneal tendon is greatly enlarged and it is difficult to discern the tendon's outer margin. The normal hyperechoic (white) densely packed fibers have been effaced by irregular hypoechoic (dark gray) areas and cavitated regions (black round areas). The soft tissues superficial to the tendon are also thickened. The sonographic diagnosis is calcaneal tendonitis with marked fiber disruption.
ii. Ultrasound of tendon injuries is useful to evaluate the extent of injury and can better characterize lesions than palpation. Performing ultrasound examinations of tendons and ligaments in small animals is difficult due to the limited size of the structures. Maintaining sufficient contact between the ultrasound transducer and the body part can be extremely difficult, and artefacts in the area immediately next to the transducer can obscure lesions and normal anatomy; however, the common calcaneal tendon in dogs can be adequately examined with ultrasound. High frequency (7.5 MHz or 10 MHz) transducers are required to obtain diagnostic images. Ultrasonographic evaluation of tendons allows differentiation between peritendinous soft tissue swelling and actual tendon enlargement. Although only transverse images are shown in this case, longitudinal plane images are also useful to detect alterations in the fine parallel arrangement of the tendon fibers and to evaluate the length of lesions. Partial or complete tears of the tendon result in varying degrees of discontinuity of the hyperechoic tendon fibers. Acute lesions are usually anechoic due to hematoma formation and edema. As lesions heal, the echogenicity of the disrupted areas gradually increases. Calcification of injured tendons occurs occasionally and will appear as hyperechoic interfaces with anechoic (black) shadows deep to the calcified areas. Serial ultrasound examinations can be used to follow the progression of tendon healing and to guide rehabilitation. Ultrasound examination of tendons and muscles is also valuable for localization of foreign bodies.

158 i. Multiple, small, well-defined lytic lesions are present in the head, neck and proximal shaft of both femurs. Similar lytic lesions are present in the pelvis and dorsal spinous processes of the lumbar vertebrae.
ii. These abnormalities are most consistent with a diagnosis of multiple myeloma. Lymphoma is another less likely differential diagnosis. Multiple myeloma is a malignant systemic tumor of plasma cells which occurs most frequently in older dogs. High levels of circulating immunoglobulins and organ infiltration by neoplastic cells can produce a wide range of clinical signs. Radiographically, the disease is associated with multiple punctate lytic lesions which most commonly affect the axial skeleton and flat bones.

159 A three-week, follow-up radiograph of an oblique radius and ulna fracture which was stabilized with a uniplanar–bilateral external skeletal fixator (159a). There is purulent drainage coming from the fixation pin tracts. Loosening and plastic deformation of fixation pins can be seen on the radiograph.
i. Discuss why the fixation method used on this dog is failing.
ii. Will the administration of antibiotics be likely to resolve this problem?
iii. Describe how management of this fracture could have been 'balanced' through a 'biologic' method of repair.

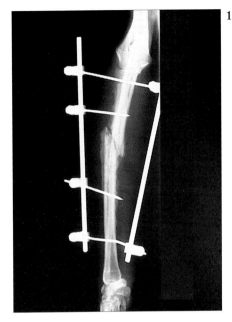
159a

160 A lateral view radiograph of the elbow of a dog which has undergone an arthrodesis using a ten-hole, 3.5 mm DCP and ten cortical bone screws (160).
i. Why was the bone plate applied to the caudal rather than the cranial aspect of the limb?
ii. What kind of orthopedic implants were used to reattach the olecranon?
iii. What angle is most commonly advocated for elbow arthrodesis?

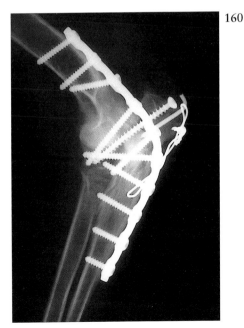
160

159 i. The oblique fracture pattern produces strong axial forces that are not being adequately controlled with this simple four pin uniplanar–bilateral frame. The axial forces produce high stress and strain, which are concentrated at the fixation pin–bone interfaces. These forces cause bone resorption and replacement with more strain tolerant fibrous tissue resulting in the fixation pins becoming loose in the bone. The movement associated with loose fixation pins is painful, resulting in high patient morbidity and delayed healing.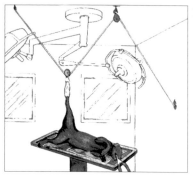

ii. Antibiotics alone are unlikely to resolve these complications. The increased inflammation and infection associated with the pin tracts are primarily the result of premature fixation pin loosening and motion. Motion at the fixation pin-bone interfaces potentiates inflammation and hinders the regional cellular response ability to control microorganisms that are constantly present in the pin tracts. Antibiotics alone will not control this infection. Primary treatment must consist of eliminating the loose fixation pin(s) and adequate stabilization of the fracture.

iii. Adequate fracture stability must be appropriately balanced with fracture healing to minimize post-operative complications. This describes the classical orthopedic race; healing must proceed rapidly enough to prevent premature loosening of implants. For this oblique fracture an external skeletal fixation configuration should have been constructed that would more efficiently resist axial loads. A type II or III configuration using six to eight appropriately inserted positive profile, partially-threaded fixation pins should have been used. If the fixator could have been applied using a closed application method, healing would proceed more rapidly than with an open application method. This 'biologic' method of application can be facilitated by hanging the limb during fixator application (**159b**).

160 i. The plate was applied in this position because the caudal aspect of the elbow is the tension surface of the joint. Stainless steel bone plates are more resistant to deformation when loaded in tension rather than in compression or bending. For that reason, application of bone plates on the tension surface decreases the probability of implant complications or failure.

ii. A cancellous bone screw, Kirschner wire and tension band wire. The olecranon osteotomy was performed to allow close contact of the plate with the caudal surface of the distal humerus and the proximal ulna.

iii. Approximately 140°. The elbow should be arthrodesed at a physiologic angle to achieve the best function possible following arthrodesis. The simplest method of determining the correct angle for an individual dog is to measure the standing angle of the elbow on the contralateral limb.

161 With regard to the dog in 160, name a potential long-term complication of elbow arthrodesis performed using a bone plate which could occur following complete and successful elbow arthrodesis, especially in an active dog.

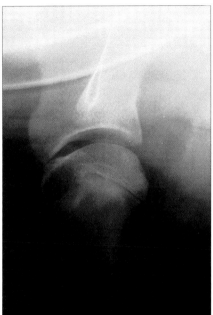

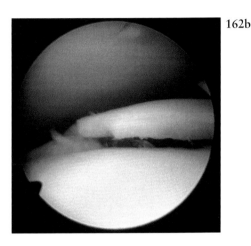

162 An extended mediolateral view radiograph (162a) and an arthroscopic view (162b) of a right scapulohumeral joint obtained from an eight-month-old, male Beauceron with an intermittent weight-bearing lameness of the right forelimb of two months' duration.
i. What is the radiographic diagnosis?
ii. Is there a correlation between the size of the radiographic lesion and the clinical abnormalities present?
iii. What is the significance of the gray line parallel to the subchondral bone of the humeral head, and what is this phenomenon called?
iv. Was arthroscopy essential for establishing a diagnosis in this dog?

161 Arthrodesis of the elbow produces a very long immobile bone segment. The ends of the plate and the most proximal and the most distal screws act as stress risers, increasing the risk of a fracture. Fracture of the humerus just proximal to the plate or a fracture of the radius and ulna just distal to the plate (as occurred in the cat in **161**) is a potential long-term complication.

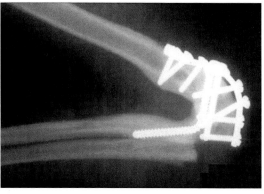

161

162 i. There is an irregular radiolucent subchondral bone defect involving the caudal aspect of the humeral head. This is the most common radiographic finding of associated osteochondrosis of the scapulohumeral joint. This lesion cannot be distinguished as an OCD lesion on plain radiographs unless the OCD cartilage flap has mineralized. Mineralized cartilage flaps are usually seen overlying the subchondral defect; however, the flap may become detached and be located elsewhere in the joint. Additional radiographic findings typically include subchondral bone sclerosis surrounding the defect and secondary degenerative joint disease in more chronic cases.
ii. Although the relationship is not absolute, larger subchondral bone lesions are more likely to be OCD lesions associated with fissuring and fragmentation of the surface of the articular cartilage and clinical signs of pain and lameness. Smaller lesions are more likely to be osteochondrosis lesions that have not penetrated the articular cartilage surface. Osteochondrosis lesions that have not disrupted the surface of the articular cartilage are not associated with overt clinical signs of pain or lameness.
iii. This finding is called the vacuum phenomenon and is caused by gas which collects in the joint space when opposing joint surfaces are physically distracted, as they are when the forelimb is placed in the extended position during radiography. Detection of the vacuum phenomenon is associated with the presence of a cartilage flap and clinical signs of pain and lameness, and an absence of joint effusion. In one study the vacuum phenomenon was observed in 20% of the scapulohumeral joints with OCD lesions.
iv. Although arthroscopy is superior to all other imaging modalities in evaluating the status of the articular cartilage and detecting joint mice, plain and contrast radiographs can usually yield comparable information. Arthroscopy does, however, allow for simultaneous diagnosis and treatment. Arthroscopic removal of a cartilage flap can be done with minimal soft tissue trauma, with a rapid return to function and minimal post-operative morbidity.

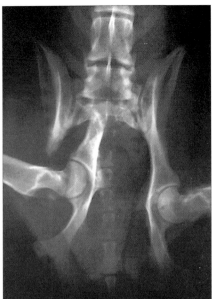

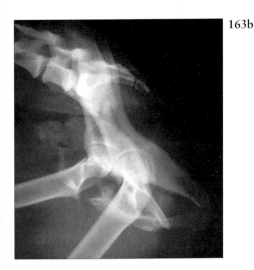

163 Ventrodorsal (163a) and lateral (163b) view pelvic radiographs of a three-year-old, female Boxer that was hit by a car.
i. Describe the fractures.
ii. Give four general indications which justify surgical intervention for pelvic fractures.
iii. Name two methods of stabilization which would be appropriate for this fracture.

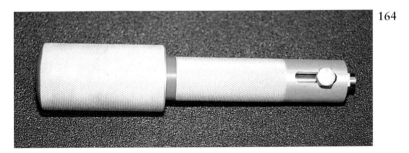

164 Name this surgical instrument (164).

163c

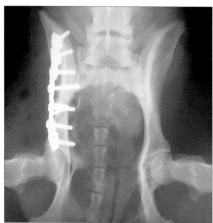

163d

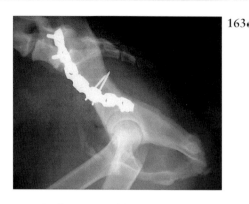

163 i. There is an oblique fracture of the right ilium with concomitant fractures of the right ischium and pubis. The acetabular segment is displaced cranially and medially.

ii. Many pelvic fractures can be managed without surgery, particularly fractures that are minimally displaced. The abundant regional musculature prevents further displacement of the fracture segments and provides an abundant blood supply to promote fracture healing. There are four general indications which may justify surgical intervention: fractures involving the acetabulum; neurologic dysfunction, most commonly ipsilateral sciatic nerve deficits; substantial compromise of the pelvic canal as determined by radiographic evaluation and rectal palpation; and an acetabular segment which is 'free floating'.

These are not absolute justifications for surgical intervention; rather each case must be evaluated individually. This dog was intended to be used as a breeding bitch and the diameter of this dog's pelvic canal was markedly decreased. Also, the concomitant fractures of the right ilium, ischium and pubis resulted in the right acetabulum segment being a 'free floating' segment which would not allow load to be transferred from the right hindlimb through the ilium to the sacrum during weight-bearing.

iii. Oblique ilial fractures can be stabilized using a bone plate placed on the lateral surface of the ilium or using lag screws placed in a ventral-to-dorsal direction. Both techniques have produced satisfactory clinical results. Although lag screw fixation of oblique ilial fractures provides superior stability to bone plates, bone plates are more commonly used to stabilize ilial fractures. Placement of lag screws in the ilium can be technically difficult, while application of plates to the lateral surface of the ilium is generally much simpler. In the example shown here, a reconstruction plate was used to stabilize the fracture (163c). The interfragmentary Kirschner wires were placed to maintain fracture reduction during bone plate application (163d).

164 IMEX tensioning device which is used to tension fixation wires during circular external skeletal fixation application.

165a

165 Craniocaudal (165a) and lateral (165b) view radiographs of the elbow of a three-month-old, male Boxer with a mild weight-bearing lameness of the right forelimb.
i. What condition is affecting this dog's elbow?
ii. What would be the appropriate treatment for this condition?

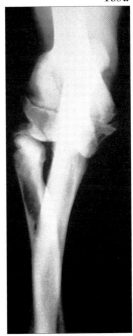

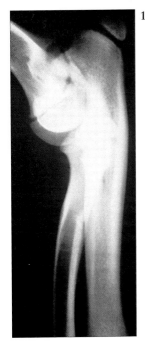

165b

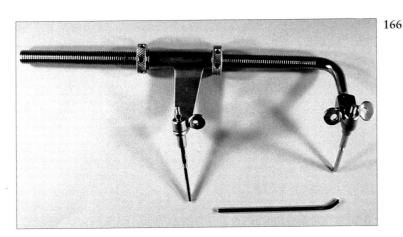

166

166 What is the instrument shown (166) and how is it applied?

165c

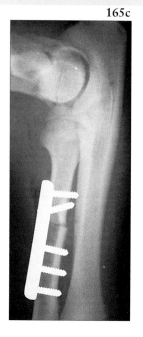

165d

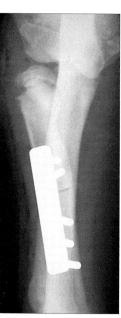

165 i. Congenital elbow luxation, which is an uncommon condition in dogs. Two types of congenital elbow luxations have been described: humeroradial luxations and humeroulnar luxations. This dog has a humeroradial luxation in which the radial head is displaced caudally, proximally and laterally. This condition is presumed to be congenital, but could be a developmental abnormality. The status of the distal radial and ulnar physes should be evaluated. Humeroradial luxations have been reported most often in large breed dogs. The condition may not always be associated with lameness. In dogs with congenital humeroulnar luxations, the ulna is usually laterally displaced, causing antebrachial rotation and marked limb deformity. Humeroulnar luxations occur most commonly in small breed dogs. It is unknown if either of these conditions have an hereditary basis.

ii. Surgical correction of this condition involves either wedge osteotomy of the proximal radius to restore congruency of the humeroradial articulation or radial head excision. In this dog a wedge osteotomy was performed and stabilized with a bone plate and screws (165c, d). Radial osteotomy generally results in improved limb function; however, in one study, radiographic follow-up showed a 30% incidence of reluxation, which was attributed to further asynchronous growth. The optimum time to perform the radial osteotomy is between four and six months of age.

166 An AO/ASIF femoral distractor. The distractor is applied by drilling holes transversely through the bone being repaired, far enough proximal and distal to the fracture so as not to interfere with application of a permanent fixation device. For a fracture near the end of a bone, the distractor may be applied spanning the adjacent joint. The connecting bolts are inserted into the holes and the fracture is distracted by turning the distracting nut on the threaded rod which forces the movable wing along the length of the threaded rod. The nut (see 167) on the opposite side of the movable wing can be used to compress fracture fragments.

167 With regard to the AO/ASIF femoral distractor illustrated in **166** and shown here in use (**167**), list five indications for the use of the instrument.

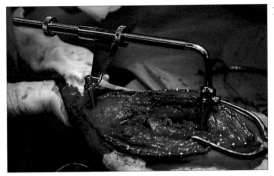

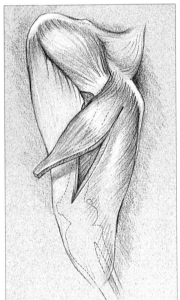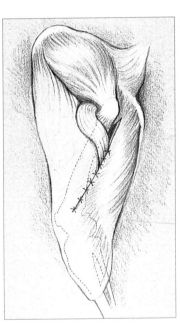

168 The biceps femoris muscle sling was developed to improve limb function in large and giant breed dogs following femoral head and neck excision. The procedure utilizes a single pedicle flap harvested from the cranial portion of the biceps femoris muscle (**168a**) which is interposed between the ostectomy site and the acetabulum (**168b**).
i. Does the biceps femoris muscle sling improve limb function following femoral head and neck incision?
ii. What morphologic changes occur in the muscle flap following dissection and transposition?

167 The AO/ASIF femoral distractor is useful for: (1) reduction of fresh diaphyseal fractures in large, well-muscled animals; (2) reduction of neglected overridden fractures; (3) bridging of joints to facilitate reduction of fractures in the metaphyseal or epiphyseal regions; (4) correction of growth disparities that require bone lengthening; (5) maintenance of the normal spatial and rotational relationships between the ends of bone segments during fitting of a cortical allograft to replace a missing diaphyseal segment.

168 i. The efficacy of the biceps femoris muscle sling remains a contentious issue. Excellent clinical results have been reported; however, the criteria used to evaluate the efficacy of the biceps femoris muscle sling in these studies were based principally on subjective assessment by owners. In addition, one clinical retrospective study (again based on subjective owner assessment) did not substantiate any improvement in limb function in dogs in which an adjunctive biceps femoris muscle sling was performed. The results of one experimental study, performed in normal dogs in which limb function was evaluated both subjectively and objectively, indicated there was no advantage in using an adjunctive biceps femoris muscle sling in comparison with femoral head and neck excision alone; however, a more recent experimental study performed in normal dogs found that dogs receiving an

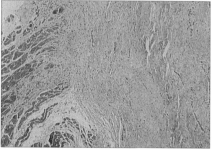

168c

168d

adjunctive partial thickness biceps femoris muscle sling had improved limb function and range of motion following femoral head and neck excision. Thus, the controversy has yet to be resolved.

ii. A substantial portion of the flap situated beneath and distal to the ostectomy site becomes infarcted and undergoes necrosis when it is placed in the former joint space (**168c**). In one experimental study it was observed that flaps that were dissected and returned to their normal anatomic position did not become infarcted. Thus infarction and necrosis were ascribed to vascular occlusion as a result of compression placed on the flap by the osteotomy site during weight-bearing. Necrosis and infarction of the flap can be associated with pyrexia, limb edema and cellulitis, as well as predisposing dogs to post-operative infection. It should also be noted that the infarcted regions of the flap are replaced with dense regular connective tissue (**168d**) and that neither early post-operative complications nor extensive fibrosis are necessarily associated with a poor final clinical outcome.

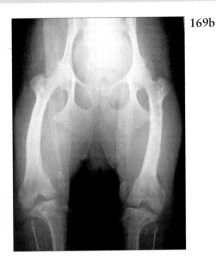

169a

169b

169 A photograph (169a) and a ventrodorsal view radiograph (169b) of the pelvis and hindlimbs of a ten-month-old, female Papillon that walks with an extremely crouched hindlimb posture. When purchased at eight weeks of age the dog was able to walk but appeared 'bow-legged'. As the dog has grown, the dog's hindlimb gait has become more crouched and the dog's mobility has decreased. Both stifles are held permanently in flexion and cannot be fully extended. Both hindpaws are internally rotated. Overt pain cannot be elicited on manipulation of the hindlimbs.
i. Describe the radiographic abnormalities.
ii. What other specific musculoskeletal abnormalities would this dog be expected to have on physical examination?

170 A ten-year-old German Shepherd Dog presented with a tumor involving the stifle joint. Radiographs revealed a proliferative and destructive process affecting both the distal femur and the proximal tibia. Biopsy and histopathologic examination of the tissue determined that the lesion was a malignant tumor. The limb was amputated and a large soft tissue mass was found destroying the bones composing the stifle joint (170).
i. What is the most likely diagnosis?
ii. What is the recommended treatment and prognosis for a dog affected with this type of tumor?

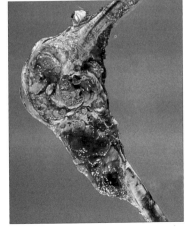

170

169 i. The abnormalities are similar in both hindlimbs. There is a bowing deformity of the femur with the distal femur bowed medially (genu varum) and hypoplasia of the medial femoral condyle. There is a medial torsional deformity of the proximal tibia of almost 90° with medial deviation of the tibial tubercle. Also present is a tilting of the transcondylar axis of the femorotibial articulation. Both patellae are positioned medial to their respective femoral condyle. The severity of the radiographic abnormalities are consistent with bilateral grade IV medial patellar luxation.

ii. The quadriceps muscle group is responsible for stifle extension and its main antagonist muscle group is the hamstring muscle group (semimembranosis, semitendinosis, biceps femoris muscles). Inability to extend the stifle may arise due to changes within the joint itself, failure of the quadriceps muscle group to extend the joint or restriction of extension caused by failure of the hamstring muscle group to relax. Palpation should include evaluation of these muscle groups and the stifle joint to ascertain the reason the stifle cannot be extended. The location of the patella and tibial tubercle should be determined, as the position of these structures in relation to the axis of the femur and tibia influence the ability of the quadriceps to extend the stifle. In this dog there is mild effusion and joint capsule thickening in both stifles and mild, generalized hindlimb muscle atrophy. The distal portion of the quadriceps muscle group deviates to the medial aspect of the limb and the patella is permanently fixed medial to the trochlear groove. The tibial tubercle is positioned on the medial side of the stifle and the distal limb rotation appears to originate at a point located just distal to the stifle.

170 i. The most common tumor that arises from the periarticular tissue is synovial cell sarcoma. Synovial cell sarcomas arise from mesenchymal precursor cells located on the periphery of the synovial membrane of joints. The radiographic finding of both a productive and destructive process affecting both the distal femur and proximal tibia is highly suggestive of this dog having a synovial cell sarcoma. There are two cell types identified within these neoplasms: an epithelioid (synovioblastic) cell type and a fibroblastic cell type. The percentage of each cell type can vary between individual tumors, which can make definitive histologic characterization of the synovial cell sarcomas difficult.

ii. Amputation of the affected limb is the recommended treatment. Disease-free intervals and survival times of more than 36 months have been reported in dogs treated by amputation alone. Clinical stage and histologic grading have been demonstrated to influence survival times. Dogs with regional lymph node or distant metastases and dogs with higher histologic grade tumors have significantly shorter survival times. Local recurrence at the amputation site has been reported and therefore amputation must be performed as proximal to the actual tumor as possible. Metastasis has been reported in as many as 41% of dogs diagnosed with synovial cell sarcoma. Adjuvant therapy has been used to prevent and treat metastatic disease but successful protocols have yet to be determined.

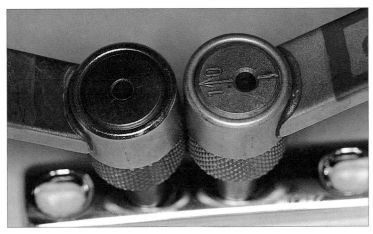

171a

171 A photograph of a 3.5 mm AO/ASIF dynamic compression bone plate and the two drill guides used for the placement of screws with this system (171a).
i. Name the two drill guides pictured.
ii. How do these drills differ with regard to drill placement within the holes in the plate?

172 A dorsopalmar view radiograph of the right carpus of a seven-year-old, male domestic shorthair cat which presented with a three-month history of lameness, weight loss and lethargy (172). On clinical examination the cat was pyrexic with bilaterally warm, swollen, painful carpi and hocks. Crepitus was elicited on manipulation of all of these joints. Significant muscle wasting was noted in both fore- and hindlimbs.
i. Describe the radiographic abnormalities.
ii. What is the most likely diagnosis?
iii. What further tests should be performed to substantiate the tentative diagnosis?

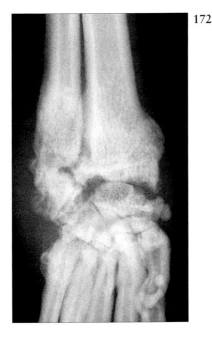

172

171 i. These are two drill guides specifically designed for use with the AO/ASIF dynamic compression plating system. The drill guide with the centrally located hole is the neutral drill guide and is coded by the 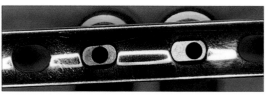 green band. The drill guide with the eccentrically located hole is the load drill guide and is coded by the yellow band (**171b**).
ii. Neutral screw placement is used when the DCP is being applied as a neutralization plate. The neutral drill guide is used to center the screw in the middle of the screw hole in the plate, thus maintaining the plate in the same position relative to the bone. Screws placed with the neutral drill guide actually impinge slightly on the sloping surface of the DCP hole near the final screw position, generating 0.1 mm displacement. Eccentric screw placement is used when dynamic compression of transverse fractures is desired. The load drill guide is designed to provide displacement of the plate relative to the bone as the screw is tightened, thereby advancing the bone segments toward each other and creating interfragmentary compression. Load drill guides are designed to provide a proportional amount of displacement depending on the plate size. 1.0 mm of bone-plate displacement is produced by the eccentric placement of a screw in a 3.5 mm DCP. This displacement can be used in an additive fashion, providing additional compression by loading sequential screws. There is, however, a maximal limit of displacement (4 mm for the 3.5 mm DCP) when two screws are placed in load fashion on each side of the fracture.

172 i. There is substantial soft tissue swelling that is most pronounced on the lateral aspect of the carpus. Periosteal new bone is visible on the styloid process of the ulna and on the medial styloid process of the radius. In both instances the new bone extends beyond the margins of the joint. The antebrachiocarpal joint space is irregularly widened and there is subchondral bone loss of the radiocarpal bone and of the distal radius. An enthesophyte is visible at the base of metacarpal bone V.
ii. The most likely diagnosis is periosteal proliferative polyarthritis. This is an immune-mediated erosive arthropathy that occurs more commonly in cats than dogs. This condition is generally bilaterally symmetrical and frequently affects the hocks and carpi. Typically, marked periosteal, periarticular new bone formation is seen radiographically. Other characteristic changes include loss of subchondral bone and enthesopathy.
iii. Synovial fluid analysis and histologic examination of the synovial membrane should be performed to establish a definitive diagnosis. The synovial fluid will typically have decreased viscosity and contain increased numbers of white blood cells, predominately polymorphonuclear cells. Histologic examination of the synovial membrane demonstrates a predominantly mononuclear cell synovitis. The disease mimics rheumatoid arthritis except that fewer joints are affected, there is extensive periarticular new bone, enthesopathy may occur and there is an absence of circulating rheumatoid factor.

173 List three potential complications or disadvantages associated with the use of the AO/ASIF femoral distractor (illustrated in 166 and 167).

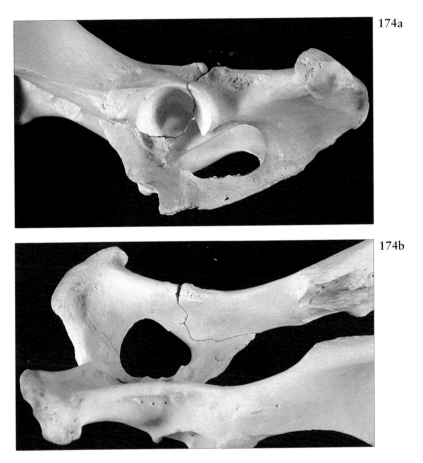

174 Photographs of a pelvis obtained from a 24-month-old racing Greyhound that became acutely lame in the left hindlimb upon accelerating out of the starting box (174a, b).
i. Describe the pathology present.
ii. What is the pathogenesis of the condition?

173 Complications or disadvantages associated with the use of the AO/ASIF femoral distractor include: (1) potential fracture of the bone through the holes drilled for the connecting bolts during the convalescent period; (2) correction of axial alignment of the fracture fragments cannot be made after distraction with the older model of the distractor (as shown in **166, 167**) without drilling new holes for the connecting bolts in a different orientation (the newer model has a double hinged connecting bolt clamp which allows angular adjustments); (3) overzealous distraction could result in damage to soft tissues; (4) in small dogs, as much as 2 cm of the connecting bolts could protrude from the *trans*-cortex of the bone into the soft tissues.

174 i. There is a minimally displaced fracture of the left acetabulum. The fracture exits dorsally through the caudal third of the acetabulum. The fracture bifurcates ventrally, extending cranioventrally through the acetabulum and into the ilium and through the caudoventral acetabulum. No other fractures of the pelvis are evident. These findings are characteristic of an acetabular stress fracture. **ii.** This type of fracture is unique to the racing Greyhound because of the tremendous repetitive stresses placed on the caudodorsal aspect of the acetabulum during racing and training. The highly developed hamstring, gluteal and external rotator muscles of the caudal thigh region produce compressive, tensile, bending and shear forces about the acetabulum during the propulsive phase of

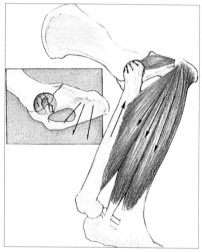

the gait. The compressive force of the femoral head acts as a fulcrum within the acetabulum while distally and laterally directed muscular forces are placed on the ischium (**174c**). The combined forces produce an area of maximum tensile and shear stresses over the caudal third of the acetabulum. When the magnitude of force produces stresses which exceed the limits of elastic deformation of the bone, plastic deformation produces microfractures of interosteonic lamellar bone. If the magnitude of physical activity remains high without allowing sufficient time for repair of these microfractures, the microfractures will coalesce, resulting in a much lower ultimate yield strain of the bone. When forces applied exceed the lowered ultimate yield strain, 'stress fractures' develop.

Acetabular stress fractures follow the primary stress riser, extending through the caudal third of the acetabulum, advancing into the acetabular fossa and splitting through the cranioventral acetabulum and caudoventrally through the acetabular incisure, producing the characteristic inverted 'Y' fracture.

175 What is the best treatment for a racing Greyhound with an acetabular stress fracture (illustrated in 174a–c)?

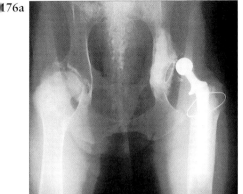

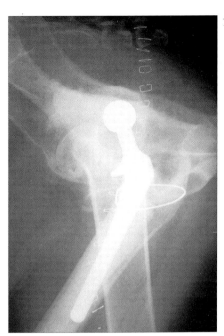

176 Immediate post-operative radiographs of a six-year-old Rottweiler that has just undergone a left total hip arthroplasty (176a, b).
i. What complication is present on these radiographs?
ii. How should this complication be initially evaluated and treated without further surgery?
iii. What surgical procedures could be done to resolve this complication if the initial non-surgical treatment failed?

175 The prognosis for successful return to competitive racing is better with surgical treatment of the fracture. In one retrospective study, only one of ten dogs treated conservatively by resting the dogs for two to six months returned to competitive racing. Surgical stabilization with dorsal acetabular plating resulted in two of two dogs treated in this manner returning to successful training and competitive racing.

176 i. The prosthetic femoral head is dislocated from the acetabular component. The acetabular component seems to be positioned properly; however, soft tissue interposition or deficit may be causing the head to dislocate. Alternatively, the femoral component may be malpositioned.
ii. Initially, an attempt should

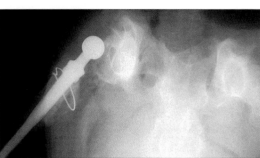
176c

be made to identify the cause of the luxation with additional radiographic views and a test closed reduction performed. To assess the open or closed position of the acetabular component a dorsal acetabular view can be obtained. This was done in this case, and positioning of the acetabular cup was acceptable (176c). The anteversion angle of the femoral component can be estimated using a true lateral radiograph of the femur and a mathematical formula. A projected anteversion angle can be measured by drawing one line through the center of the shaft of the femoral component and a second line through the mid-points of the femoral neck and head. This is corrected to the true anteversion angle by the following formula:

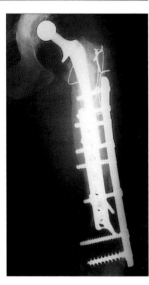
176d

$$\text{Tangent of true anterversion angle} = \frac{\text{Tangent of projected angle}}{0.707}$$

The true femoral anteversion angle was calculated to be 50° in this dog. A trial coxofemoral reduction was only stable when the femur was maximally internally rotated. This dog's luxation was reduced (closed) and the limb was in placed in a Ehmer sling for four weeks. Four months following surgery, however, the luxation recurred.
iii. Either the femoral component should be revised and repositioned or a rotational osteotomy of the femur should be considered. In this dog, a rotational osteotomy of the femur was performed to correct the excessive femoral anteversion (176d). This procedure was effective in keeping the femoral prosthesis from reluxating.

177a

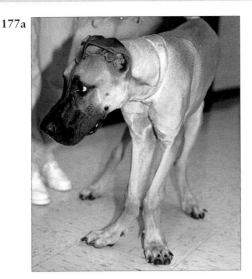

177b

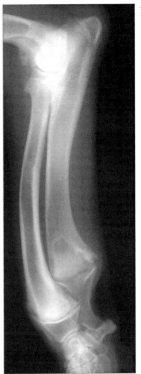

177 A photograph (177a) and lateral view radiograph (177b) of the antebrachium of a seven-month-old Great Dane that received excessive calcium supplementation. Breeders often advocate dietary calcium supplementation for growing puppies, particularly large and giant breed dogs.

i. What effect does increased dietary supplementation have on plasma calcium and phosphorous levels?

ii. What detrimental clinical effects can result from excessive dietary calcium supplementation?

178 Name this surgical implant (178).

178

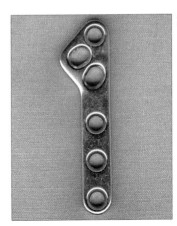

177 i. Feeding Great Dane puppies a normal diet supplemented with three times the National Research Council's recommended calcium content resulted in mild hypercalcemia with concomitant hypophosphatemia. Intestinal calcium absorption occurs by both transcellular and paracellular pathways. The transcellular pathway involves an active transport mechanism for calcium through the cell and ejection by an ATP-ase dependent calcium-pump from the basal membrane into the circulatory system. Passive calcium absorption occurs via the paracellular pathway, especially under conditions of high intraluminal calcium concentration. Intestinal excretion of calcium is independent of dietary calcium content and plays a minor role in corporeal calcium kinetics.

There is an obligatory increase in total calcium absorption as a result of increased passive absorption in dogs fed high calcium diets. High intraluminal calcium concentration also binds phosphate, preventing phosphate absorption. In addition, the resultant hypercalcemia is associated with a concomitant hypophosphatemia as an inverse relationship between serum calcium and phosphorus levels exist. This hypophosphatemia is less profound when both calcium and phosphorus intake is excessive.

The increased calcium absorption decreases parathyroid hormone secretion, decreasing renal calcium reabsorption and osteoclasia. Renal conversion of 25-OH_2 vitamin D to $1,25\text{-OH}_2$ vitamin D, the most active metabolite which activates osteoclasts, stimulates renal reabsorption of calcium and phosphorus, and increases active intestinal absorption of calcium and decreases phosphorus reabsorption. High calcium intake stimulates calcitonin secretion, which prevents osteoclasia and thus release of calcium from the skeletal system.

These hormonal influences result in net deposition of calcium in the skeletal system as osteoblastic activity is increased and osteoclastic activity is decreased, which mitigates elevations in plasma calcium concentration. Thus, there is not a direct correlation between calcium and phosphorus consumption and plasma calcium and phosphorous concentrations.
ii. Skeletal abnormalities in Great Dane puppies which received excessive dietary calcium were characterized by decreased osteoclastic activity and thus increased total bone volume and retarded bone remodeling causing cervical vertebral malformation and panosteitis. In addition, disturbances in enchondral ossification of both articular and physeal cartilage resulted in stunted growth, osteochondrosis of multiple joints and RCCs in the distal ulna causing radius curvis syndrome as occurred in this dog (177b). Large and giant breed dogs seem to be particularly susceptible to developing skeletal abnormalities when fed diets containing excess calcium. Miniature Poodles fed high calcium diets did not develop similar abnormalities.

178 A Slocum tibial plateau leveling osteotomy plate. This plate is used to stabilize the tibial plateau segment which is rotated caudally during the tibial plateau leveling osteotomy for the treatment of CCL injuries in dogs.

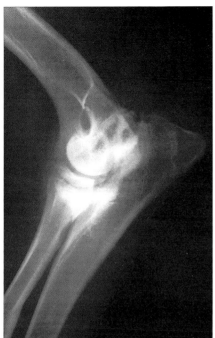

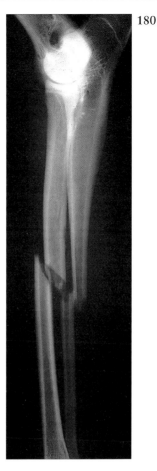

179 A lateral view radiograph of the left elbow of a five-month-old Irish Wolfhound with a left forelimb lameness of four weeks' duration (**179**).
i. Describe the radiographic abnormalities.
ii. List three treatment options for this condition.

180 A lateral view radiograph of the antebrachium of a Grade A racing Greyhound that sustained closed oblique fractures of the radius and ulna during a racing altercation with another dog (**180**).

How would appropriate treatment of this fracture differ in a racing Greyhound as compared with a dog that was a pet?

183

179 i. The radial head is subluxated proximally and the anconeal process has failed to unite with the ulna. There are early degenerative changes present in the elbow.

ii. (1) Excision of the united anconeal process has been, and remains, the most common treatment for ununited anconeal process. Although degenerative changes continue to progress in the affected elbow following process excision, most dogs obtain surprisingly good limb function. In one study evaluating the results of anconeal process excision, 16 dogs (19 elbows) were evaluated with the follow-up mean time being 19.5 months after surgery. All dogs had crepitus and decreased range of motion in the affected elbow(s); however, none of the dogs exhibited overt lameness on the affected limb(s). (2) Lag screw fixation of the united anconeal process. Although stabilization of the ununited anconeal process using lag screw fixation has been purported to be associated with numerous technical complications and to be of questionable value, a recent study reported radiographic union of the ununited anconeal process following lag screw stabilization in five of six elbows available for follow-up evaluation. Unfortunately, details regarding elbow and limb function were not included. (3) Proximal diaphyseal ulnar osteotomy. Elbow incongruity, specifically proximal subluxation of the radial head, exerts abnormal stress on the developing anconeal process indirectly via the humeral condyle which results in failure of the process to fuse with the ulna. In a recent study, 15 of 17 dogs unilaterally affected with ununited anconeal processes had proximal displacement of the radial head in the affected elbow. Proximal diaphyseal ulnar osteotomy is performed to restore congruency of the elbow, thereby relieving the abnormal load on the anconeal process. In the above study the anconeal process fused in 21 of 22 elbows treated in this manner and limb function was generally favorable. This procedure is probably most efficacious in young dogs. Whether restoration of congruency improves elbow function in association with process excision or lag screw fixation in older dogs has yet to be established.

180 The treatment options with a pet dog would include external coaptation, external skeletal fixation and open reduction and internal fixation with plates and screws. When treating a performance animal such as a racing Greyhound, primary bone union that results from rigid fixation is a desirable outcome. The absence of a large bony callus prevents interference with muscles and tendons; however, it is generally recognized that many internal fixation devices need to be removed prior to resumption of competitive activities.

181 With regard to the racing Greyhound in 180, describe a treatment protocol that will return the dog to competitive racing within 16–20 weeks.

182 Post-operative craniocaudal (182a) and lateral (182a, b) view radiographs of a comminuted mid-diaphyseal tibial fracture which was stabilized with an interlocking intramedullary nail.
i. Define the term interfragmentary strain.
ii. What are the approximate interfragmentary strain environments which bone, cartilage and granulation tissue can tolerate?

182a
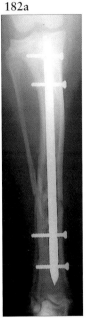

182b
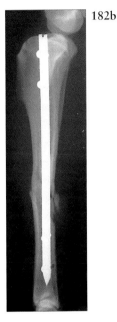

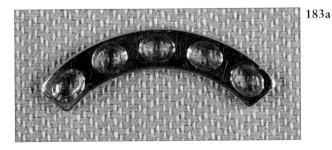
183a

183 A photograph of an implant used commonly in veterinary orthopedic surgery (183a).
i. What is the name of this implant?
ii. What is the purported advantage for the use of this implant?

181 The radial fracture is approached through a craniomedial incision and the fracture is anatomically reduced and stabilized with an appropriately sized (2.7 or 3.5 mm) DCP placed on the medial surface of the radius. Interfragmentary compression of the fracture fragments is done when possible. Limitation of full carpal flexion may occur due to distraction of the fracture segments unless the ulna is also stabilized. Consequently, the ulnar fracture is approached through a lateral incision, reduced and stabilized with either a 2.0 mm DCP or a 2.7/2.0 veterinary cuttable plate. A Robert Jones bandage is applied for one week, and radiographs are obtained at four and eight weeks following surgery. Cortical and medullary continuity is used to evaluate radiographic union because it is difficult to radiographically assess fracture healing during primary bone union. Frequently, Greyhounds treated in this manner achieve union by eight weeks. Both plates are removed at this time, and leash restriction is instituted for approximately four weeks. Radiographs are again obtained to assess bone ingrowth into the screw holes. Limited training activities are discussed and, hopefully, full activity can be reinstated by 16 weeks.

182 i. When axial loads are applied to a structure it undergoes deformation resulting in the generation of internal forces. The intensity of these forces is referred to as internal stresses and the deformations as internal strains. Similarly, when a load is applied to a fractured bone, strain is produced at the fracture site which is referred to as interfragmentary strain. Interfragmentary strain can be calculated as a ratio of the change in length divided by the original length of the fracture gap. For example, if a 3 mm fracture gap is compressed 1 mm during loading, the interfragmentary strain is one divided by three, i.e. 33%. Interfragmentary strain can be minimized by providing rigid fixation (decreasing the change in length) or by avoiding anatomic reconstruction of fracture fragments (yielding a greater original length).
ii. The fate of interfragmentary tissues is strongly affected by the local strain environment. Granulation tissue can tolerate a local strain environment up to 100%, cartilage up to 10% and bone approximately 2%. In fracture gaps with strain levels less than 2%, undifferentiated cells differentiate into osteoblasts and produce bone. In higher strain environments, cellular differentiation favors osteoclasis and chondrogenesis or fibrogenesis. A clinical example of the importance of interfragmentary strain is the widening of fracture gaps often seen on radiographs obtained several weeks after a fracture has been repaired. If the original fracture gap was 5 mm and the gap displaced 1 mm when loaded, bone at the ends of the fracture segments will be resorbed and the fracture gap will widen, as bone is unable to survive in a 20% strain environment. This resorption of bone at the fracture ends results in a greater 'original length', of say 10 mm. Once the gap has widened to 10 mm and the interfragmentary strain decreased to 10%, cartilage can proliferate and contribute to stability, ultimately leading to a strain environment conducive to bone formation and fracture union.

183 i. A 5-hole, 2.7 mm AO/ASIF veterinary acetabular plate. A 2.0 mm veterinary acetabular plate which accepts six 2.0 mm cortical screws is also available.
ii. Veterinary acetabular plates were specifically designed for stabilization of acetabular

183b

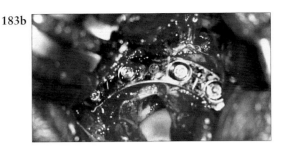

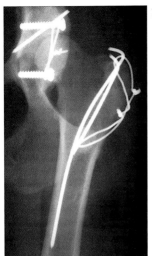
183c

fractures in dogs. The curvilinear shape of the plate simplifies contouring the plate to the dorsal acetabular surface which facilitates accurate reduction of acetabular fractures (183b). Veterinary acetabular plates are more rigid than many of the other plates which have been used for acetabular fracture repair, such as small fragment plates, mini-DCPs, finger plates and reconstruction plates. The 2.0 mm veterinary acetabular plate is used most frequently, even in relatively large dogs, because its small size allows a greater latitude in positioning the plate with respect to fracture line orientation(s) when compared with the 2.7 mm veterinary acetabular plate. Relatively small implants can be used for acetabular fracture stabilization because the implants are placed on the tensile surface of the acetabulum. Veterinary acetabular plates have been used for repair of acetabular fractures by many surgeons with very good results, particularly if there are not multiple concurrent orthopedic injuries. Despite their unique design, veterinary acetabular plates can be difficult to contour precisely to the dorsal acetabular surface and thus anatomic fracture reduction may not be achieved.

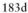
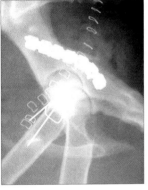
183d

Another method of acetabular fracture repair which results in significantly better reduction of the articular surface involves the placement of an interfragmentary Kirschner wire(s), bone screws in the cranial and caudal fracture segments, and a figure-of-eight tension band wire between the screws to compress and stabilize the fracture. PMMA bone cement is molded over the screws and figure-of-eight wire to increase implant rigidity (183c). This method of fixation has been shown to provide comparable rigidity to 2.0 mm veterinary acetabular plates and has proven successful in a large number of dogs with acetabular fractures.

Reconstruction plates are also an option for acetabular fracture stabilization in dogs and have the advantage of being easily contoured in three planes (183d). Reconstruction plates are also available in lengths sufficient to allow ipsilateral pelvic fractures (e.g. ilial and acetabular) to be stabilized with a single, properly contoured plate.

Index

Degenerative joint disease (*continued*)
  osteochondrosis/OCD 120, 131, 162
  PSGAG treatment 14
  synovial fluid 135
  triple pelvic osteotomy 72
Demodicosis 19
Dental composite 9
Dermatomyositis 19
Desmotomy 29
DeVita pin 73
Dirofilariasis 121
Discospondylitis 63, 64
Distraction index 5
Distraction osteogenesis 74
Disuse osteopenia 130
Drill guides 171
Dynamic compression plate (DCP) 39, 91, 183
  arthrodesis 160
  displacement maximal limit 171
  femoral fracture 104, 139
  interlocking nail fixation 84
  materials 119
  radial fracture 181

Ehmer sling 149, 176
Ehrlichia spp. 1
Elbow joint
  arthrodesis 160, 161
  congenital luxation 165
  fragmented coronoid process 29, 154, 155
  osteochondritis dissecans 29
  traumatic luxation 95
  ununited anconeal process 179
Electromyography 19
Elution properties 49
Endrochondral ossification 131
Enophthalmos 70
Enthesopathy 172
Epiphyseal growth plate 24
Escherichia coli 64, 156
Excision arthroplasty, failed 45
Exophthalmos 70
External (skeletal) fixator 8, 15, 118, 134, 164, 180
  arthrodesis 144
  acrylic connecting column 61
  adjunctive 106, 113
  bilateral 78
  complications 43, 159
  corrective osteotomy 145

External (skeletal) fixator (*continued*)
  osteotomy stabilization 66
External fixation pins 35

Facetectomy 40
Fasciotomy 17
Fat graft, autogenous 20
Femoral fracture 17, 27, 98, 104, 139, 145
  greater trochanter 30, 79
  gunshot injury 104
  non-union 15, 16, 129
  pathologic 88
  supracondylar 91
  transverse 106
Femoral head and neck excision 168
Femoral neck lengthening 76
Femoral stem implantation 142
Femur
  osteosarcoma 88
  quadriceps tie-down 21
Fibrogenesis 182
Fibroplasia 116, 124
Fibrosarcoma 69, 96
Fibrous dysplasia 96
Fibula segmental fracture 8
Fibular head transposition 110
Fistulogram 80
Flexion splint (90-90) 97
Flexor tendon disruption 4
Fluorescent rings 111
Fluorochrome labels 111
Fracture repair 15, 16, 98, 159
  interfragmentary compression 27, 118, 181
  interlocking nail fixation 84
Freer periosteal elevator 117
Fungal infection 11

Gait analysis 102
Gelpi retractors 138
Giant cell sarcoma 69
Gigli wire bone saw 127
Glenoid dysplasia 45
Glycocalyx 23
Golgi apparatus 152
Gracilis muscle avulsion 93, 94
Graft
  intra-articular 38
  isometric tensioning 38
  see also Cancellous bone, graft
Ground reaction forces 102
Gunshot injury 104

Haversian canals/systems 68, 111
Heartworm disease 1
Hemangioma 96
Hemangiosarcoma 69, 96
Hemarthrosis 14
Hepatic adenocarcinoma 121
Hip dysplasia 5, 54, 72, 149, 153
Hohmann retractor 143
Hook plate 104
Howship's lacunae 152
Humerus
    fracture 25, 26, 28, 113, 118, 125
    osteochronditis dissecans 131
    osteomyelitis 52
Hypercalcemia 177
Hyperparathyroidism 90
Hypertrophic osteodystrophy 12
Hypertrophic osteopathy 12, 121, 122
Hypophosphatemia 177
Hypothyroidism 101
Hypovitaminosis C 12

Ilizarov method 74
IMEX tensioning device 164
Incomplete ossification 25, 26
Inflammatory joint disease 1
Infraspinatus muscle contracture 132
Interfragmentary compression 27, 118, 181
Interfragmentary strain 98, 182
Interlocking nail fixation 84
Intermittent open mouth locking 92
Internal fixation 147, 180
    see also Plate; Screws
Intra-articular graft 38
Intramembranous ossification 34, 74
Ischio-ilial pin 73
Isometric tensioning 38

Jacob's hand chuck 36
Joint mouse 114, 162

Lamellae 68
Laminectomy 40
L-carnitine 87
Legg–Calvé–Perthes disease 149
Lengthening plates 139
Limb-sparing surgery 55, 56
Load sharing 8
Load/deformation curve 3
Lubra plates 148
Lymphoma 158

Mandible
    craniomandibular osteopathy 81, 82
    fracture 9, 10, 13, 43, 134
Mandibulectomy 134
Mason-meta splint 130
Maxilla fracture 61
Medullary reaming 142
Meniscectomy 14, 143
Metastatic neoplasia 11
Metatarsal bone stress fracture 32
Monkey muscle 37
Monteggia lesion 150, 151
Multiple myeloma 158
Muscle biopsy 42, 70, 87
Myalgia 42
Myopathy 47
    endocrine-related 101
    lipid storage 87
Myositis 70
Myotenotomy 76

Neoplasia 63, 69, 121
Neurogenic atrophy 70
Non-steroidal anti-inflammatory drugs 47
Non-union
    secondary to implant failure 108, 125
    fracture 129
Norberg angle 5
Nutritional secondary
    hyperparathyroidism 90

Orthopedic Foundation for Animals 5
Ortolani sign 54, 72
Oscillating saw 145
Ossification
    incomplete 25, 26
    intramembranous 34, 74
Ostectomy 20, 92, 168
Osteoarthritis 38, 53, 58, 116
Osteoblast 152
Osteochondritis dissecans 29, 114, 120, 131, 162
Osteochondroma 46
Osteochondrosis 53, 120, 131, 162, 177
Osteoclasis 182
Osteoclast 152
Osteodystrophy, hypertrophic 12
Osteogenesis 131
    distraction 74
Osteomyelitis 11, 15, 23, 48, 52, 63, 96
Osteonecrosis 124